Coroners' Rules and Statutes

by

Giles Kavanagh, M.A., LL.M.(Cantab.)
of the Middle Temple, Barrister

LONDON
SWEET & MAXWELL
1985

Published in 1985 by
Sweet & Maxwell Limited of
11, New Fetter Lane, London.
Computerset by Burgess & Son (Abingdon) Limited.
Printed in Scotland.

British Library Cataloguing in Publication Data

Coroners rules and statutes.
1. Coroners—England
I. Kavanagh, Giles
344.207′16   KD7296.A3

ISBN 0-421-33880-6

82429

For Mum and Dad

PREFACE

This is a practitioners' guide to the procedural and substantive law which regulates the powers and duties of coroners in England and Wales. Its presentation is designed to assist rapid search and location of the relevant coroners' rules and statutes.

The procedure section sets out each step to be taken before, during and after an inquest, referring the reader to the appropriate rules, forms and statutes which appear in full later in the book and to the relevant case law which appears in the footnotes to each page.

I have included the procedural guide to Appeal from and Judicial Review of coroners' decisions together with information on the use in other proceedings of evidence adduced at inquests to assist those for whom matters do not end at the door of the coroner's court.

The statutes are in keeping with the Sweet and Maxwell house style with amendments and repeals detailed in a commentary which follows each section.

These features, combined with the summary of recent developments and a thorough index, should provide the experienced and inexperienced alike with a manageable guide to coroners' proceedings.

There are four people in particular whose help I would like to acknowledge. My thanks to Robert Webb for giving me the idea for the book; Margaret Wakefield-Richmond for her considerable work in correcting and commenting on the proofs at each stage; Dr. John Burton for his advice on content; lastly, special thanks to Penelope Evans for her practical and moral support throughout.

Giles Kavanagh

1 Harcourt Buildings,
Temple,
London EC4.
May 1985

CONTENTS

TABLE OF CASES

TABLE OF STATUTES

*[Page numbers in **bold** type indicate where the statutory material referred to is set out in full.]*

TABLE OF STATUTORY INSTRUMENTS

*[Page numbers in **bold** type indicate where the statutory material referred to is set out in full.]*

RECENT DEVELOPMENTS IN CORONERS' LAW

RECENT DEVELOPMENTS IN CORONERS' LAW

RULES

The 1984 Coroners Rules became operative on July 1, 1984 consolidating the 1953 Rules as amended and effecting a number of changes of varying significance.

Adjournments—interim certificate of the fact of death

Rule 30 is new and envisages the situation where a coroner adjourns an inquest and is unable to furnish the Registrar of Deaths with a certificate stating the particulars which are required to be registered concerning the death. Upon application by an interested party the coroner is now obliged to issue an "interim certificate of the fact of death" (Form 14). This sensible provision means that the arrangement of some of the deceased's financial affairs and the administration of the estate can proceed without delay. Insurance companies will usually await the final determination of the cause of death before settling claims concerning the deceased.

Verdicts

Note 4 to the Form of Inquisition (Form 22) advises that the words "and the cause of death was aggravated by lack of care/self neglect" may only be added to the verdict, where appropriate, when the cause of death is natural or from a specific industrial disease, or from want of attention at birth or from dependence on drugs/non-dependent abuse of drugs (but see the unreported case of *Michael Martin dec'd.*, at p. 74, *post*). Rule 43 of the new Rules does permit the coroner to announce the fact that he is reporting a matter in writing to a person or authority who may have power to act where he believes that action should be taken to prevent further fatalities similar to that in respect of which the inquest is being held. Such announcements and reports do not of course form part of the verdict.

The verdict of death from chronic alcoholism does not appear in the list of verdicts in the 1984 Form of Inquisition. Before July 1, 1984 all deaths associated with chronic alcoholism were reported to the coroner. An inquest should not now be necessary in such cases unless the death is reportable on any other ground.

STATUTES

Criminal jurisdiction

The Criminal Law Act 1977 effected substantial reform in abolishing the criminal jurisdiction of the Coroner's Court. The verdicts of murder,

3

manslaughter and infanticide have been replaced by "killed unlawfully," and a coroner can no longer commit for trial nor can the jury find a named person guilty of causing the death.

The body

The Coroners Act 1980 made three changes: it abolished the legal necessity for the coroner to view the body; it provided for inquests to be held in districts other than that in which the body lies, and conferred new powers for the exhumation of bodies.

Juries

Section 62 of the Administration of Justice Act 1982, amended section 13(2) of the Coroners (Amendment) Act 1926, to require a coroner to summon a jury where the deceased died in police custody, or death resulted from an injury caused by a police officer in the purported execution of his duty.

The Coroners' Juries Act 1983 added a new section 3A to The Coroners Act 1887. In doing so it altered the qualifications for service on Coroners Courts' juries bringing them into line with the Crown Court, High Court and County Court requirements as specified in section 1 of the Juries Act 1974. Criminal penalties were provided for evading jury service and section 26 of the Coroners (Amendment) Act 1926 was amended to provide for rules to permit exemption from jury service in circumstances prescribed by those rules.[1]

CASE LAW

Jurisdiction

R. v. West Yorkshire Coroner, ex parte Smith [1982] 3 W.L.R. 920: The Court of Appeal held that when a coroner was informed that a dead body was lying within his geographical area of jurisdiction and there was reasonable cause to suspect that the death fell into one of the categories specified in section 3 of the Coroners Act 1887, he was required to hold an inquest whether the cause of death arose within his jurisdiction or not, even if it occurred outside England and Wales.

High Court—power to delete rider

R. v. Walthamstow Coroner, ex parte Rubenstein [1982] Crim L.R. 509, D.C.: Where an application was brought under the general common law a rider could be amended, deleting words, but where the application to quash was brought under section 6 of the 1887 Act, a High Court judge had no

[1] Now the Coroner's Rules 1984.

such power. He could only quash an inquisition and order a fresh inquest, where appropriate.

Jury's deliberation and verdict

Re Inquest into the death of Roberto Calvi, Dec'd., The Times, April 2, 1983: The Divisional Court, the Lord Chief Justice presiding, held that where the inquest had taken place on a single day and the jury had heard the evidence of 35 witnesses and had been sent out to consider their verdict 10 hours and 20 minutes after the hearing began, returning at 10 p.m. to deliver a majority verdict; (*a*) that was too late an hour for a jury to be considering their verdict, given that some of the evidence involved expert scientific testimony, and (*b*) the coroner's direction to the jury that an open verdict "might seem like a super open door to scuttle through" in the event of their being unable to decide in favour of either suicide or unlawful killing, implied that there was something cowardly in reaching an open verdict. The inquisition was quashed and a new inquest ordered before a different coroner.

Verdict—whether determining civil liability

R. v. *Walthamstow Coroner, ex parte Rubenstein* [1982] Crim L.R. 509, D.C.: A verdict which included the words "aggravated by neglect" was a verdict which could be reached without breach of r.33 of the 1953 Rules (now r.42, 1984 Rules, *post*) as it did not specifically refer to a particular person (*R.* v. *Surrey Coroner, ex parte Campbell* [1982] Q.B. 661, where it was held that a verdict of lack of care by another or others did not transgress the requirement under r.33, considered).

Coroner's discretion—choice of venue

R. v. *Inner North London Coroner, ex parte GLC, The Times,* April 30, 1983, Woolf J.: On application by the coroner for judicial review for a declaration, the High Court held that section 78 of the London Government Act 1963 was not intended to give the GLC power to interfere in a coroner's discretion under section 3 of the Coroners Act 1887 to specify the venue for an inquest.

Contempt—coroner's power to fine and commit

Re A.S. Rayan, The Times, October 20, 1983, Kerr J.: A coroner fined a doctor for contempt when the doctor, who had been orally summoned, appeared late for the inquest. It was held by the Divisional Court that there was no contempt and, further, as he had not been duly summoned the coroner could not fine him.

R. v. *West Yorkshire Coroner, ex parte Smith, The Times,* October 3, 1984, D.C. [C.J.]: Held, that a coroner's court is an inferior court of record, and has power to [fine and] commit for contempt (*Att.-Gen.* v. *B.B.C.* [1981] A.C. 303; [1980] 3 All E.R. 161, considered). See the Contempt of Court Act, 1981, section 14(1), (2).

Judicial review—the scope of

R. v. *Greater Manchester Coroner, ex parte Tal* [1984] 3 All E.R. 240, D.C. The Divisional Court held that the *Anisminic* principle applied to a Coroner's Court and therefore an inquest was fully subject to judicial review. In so deciding the Court disagreed with the Divisional Court decision in *R.* v. *Surrey Coroner, ex parte Campbell* [1982] Q.B. 661 that, because a Coroner's Court was a court of record, the *Anisminic* principle did not apply and judicial review could only be ordered where there was an error on the face of the inquisition, fraud or an excess or refusal of jurisdiction.

Awarding costs against coroners

R. v. *West Yorkshire Coroner, ex parte Kenyon, The Times,* April 11, 1984, D.C. [C.J.]: Where a coroner, as with any public body, did not appear and was not represented, and an error of law was not grave, costs would not be awarded against the coroner or public body.

Bias—the test

R. v. *West Yorkshire Coroner, ex parte Smith, The Times,* November 6, 1982, *per* Webster J.: Where S sought orders of prohibition and mandamus, alleging that the West Yorkshire Coroner might be biased. Held, dismissing the application, that (1) the test for these purposes would be what a reasonable man might think; (2) the appropriate time for the test was the time of the hearing which was sought to be reviewed; (3) a reasonable man should be taken to know all the matters in evidence at the hearing.

PROCEDURE

PRE-INQUEST PROCEDURE
INQUEST PROCEDURE
POST-INQUEST PROCEDURE—APPEAL
USE OF EVIDENCE ADDUCED IN SUBSEQUENT PROCEEDINGS

PROCEDURE

PRE-INQUEST PROCEDURE

	RULE (The Coroners Rules 1984)	FORM (The Coroners Rules 1984, Schedule 4)
1. Body lying within the coroner's geographical jurisdiction in circumstances which may require an inquest *i.e.* if there is reason to believe that death was due to violence or was unnatural or a sudden death of unknown cause, or took place in circumstances requiring an inquest under any Act.[1] Coroner decides whether he has jurisdiction.[2] (See note 1 for the other circumstances in which the coroner is required to exercise his judicial powers of inquiry.)		
2. Coroner may decide that it is expedient to transfer jurisdiction to a coroner in another area.[3]		
3. In certain circumstances the coroner may order exhumation of the body.[4]		2

4. The "attending registered medical practitioner": procedure:

(1) *The attending R.M.P.:*

"In the case of the death of any person who has been attended during his last illness by a registered medical practitioner, that practitioner

---

[1] Coroners Act 1887, s.3(1), *post* at p. 80. Note that the death need not have occurred within the coroner's jurisdiction, or even within England and Wales: *R.* v. *West Yorkshire Coroner, ex parte Smith* [1982] 3 W.L.R. 920.

The coroner is also required to exercise his judicial powers of inquiry in the following circumstances: when a death has been referred to him under the Registration of Births, Deaths and Marriages Regulations 1968, reg. 51; where he has reason to believe that a death has occurred in or near his jurisdiction in such circumstances that an inquest ought to be held, but the body has been destroyed or cannot be recovered and the Secretary of State directs that an inquest be held (Coroners (Amendment) Act 1926, s.18, *post* at p. 110); when jurisdiction has been transferred to him under the Coroners Act 1980, s.2; when ordered to do so by the High Court under the Coroners Act 1887, s.6, or by the Divisional Court by way of a judicial review; when it is sought to remove a body out of England; when the coroner has reason to believe that treasure has been found (see p. 96, *post*).

[2] The case may be one in which diplomatic immunity or immunity by virtue of the Visiting Forces Act 1952 applies. If so the coroner has no jurisdiction unless in the latter case directed by the Secretary of State to hold an inquest: Visiting Forces Act 1952, s.7(2) or (3).

[3] The Coroners Act 1980, s.2 empowers a coroner to do so without transferring the body.

[4] Coroners Act 1980, s.4, *post* at p. 124.

9

	RULE (The Coroners Rules 1984)	FORM (The Coroners Rules 1984, Schedule 4)

shall sign a certificate in the prescribed form stating to the best of his knowledge and belief the cause of death and shall forthwith deliver that certificate to the registrar."[5]

(2) *The Registrar:*

Either

(a) Registrar registers the cause of death shown in the certificate thereby disposing of the case

Or

(b) If the death is one:

   (i) in respect of which the deceased was not attended during his last illness by a medical practitioner; or

   (ii) in respect of which the registrar has been unable to obtain a duly completed certificate of cause of death; or

   (iii) with respect to which it appears to the registrar, from the particulars contained in such a certificate or otherwise, that the deceased was seen by the certifying medical practitioner neither after death nor within 14 days before death; or

   (iv) the cause of which appears to be unknown; or

   (v) which the registrar has reason to believe to have been unnatural or to have been caused by violence or neglect, or by abortion, or to have been attended by suspicious circumstances; or

   (vi) which appears to the registrar to have occurred during an operation or before recovery from the effect of an anaesthetic; or

[5] Births and Deaths Registration Act 1953, s.22(1).

10

	RULE (The Coroners Rules 1984)	FORM (The Coroners Rules 1984, Schedule 4)
(vii) which appears to the registrar from the contents of any medical certificate to have been due to industrial disease or industrial poisoning.[6]		

the registrar refers the death to the coroner.

(3) *The coroner:*

If the registrar refers the death to the coroner who has jurisdiction
Then
(*a*) If the coroner is satisfied:

    (i) that the deceased was attended during his last illness by a registered medical practitioner; and

    (ii) that the cause of death is natural; the coroner completes Pink Form "A" and sends it with the medical certificate of cause of death to the registrar. (The coroner uses Pink Form "A" when he has decided not to hold an inquest.)

Or
(*b*) If the coroner is not satisfied of both (i) and (ii) of (*a*) above he will EITHER hold an inquest usually, though not always, preceded by a post-mortem,[7]

	RULE	FORM
OR **5.** If no registered medical practitioner is able to give a medical certificate of the cause of death, or the death was a sudden one of unknown cause, the coroner, if he thinks that a post-mortem examination will show the cause of death to have been a natural one, may request a suitably qualified medical practitioner[8] to make a post-mortem examination.[9]	6	10

[6] Registration of Births, Deaths and Marriages Regulations 1968 (S.I. 1968 No. 2049), reg. 51.

[7] While it is nowadays usual to have a post-mortem in such cases, it is not obligatory. A very small proportion of inquests is held without post-mortem examination (usually because it would be nugatory—as with a body long submerged in water, or dangerous, *e.g.* death from lassa fever, etc.)

[8] Coroners (Amendment) Act 1926, s.22, *post*, at p. 115 for definition.

[9] *Ibid.* s.21, *post*, at p. 114. If the cause of death is shown to be natural the coroner disposes of the case using Pink Form "B" (*post*, at p. 29).

11

	RULE (The Coroners Rules 1984)	FORM (The Coroners Rules 1984, Schedule 4)
6. Coroner may either direct or request a post-mortem examination to be held because the cause of death is one which necessitates an inquest.[10]		
7. Post-mortem examination		
(1) Pathologist (or other suitably qualified medical practitioner) carries out the post-mortem by the direction or at the request of the coroner.		
(2) Certain persons or bodies are entitled to be notified by the coroner of the post-mortem examination are also entitled to be represented at such examination by a registered medical practitioner.	7	
(3) Persons attending the post-mortem by virtue of rule 7 are not to interfere with the performance of the examination.	8	
(4) The post-mortem shall be made in premises which are adequately equipped for the purpose of the examination, *i.e.* premises which have running water, proper heating and lighting facilities and containers for the storing and preservation of material.	11	
(5) The person making the post-mortem examination shall endeavour to preserve relevant material for as long as the coroner thinks fit and shall report to the coroner and shall not supply a copy of such report to any person other than the coroner unless the latter so authorises.	9 10	Sched. 2
8. Special examination		
(1) The coroner may request any legally qualified medical practitioner to carry out a special examination by way of analysis, etc.[11]		

---

[10] (*a*) See n. 7, *ante*. When the coroner has decided to hold an inquest he may request any legally qualified medical practitioner to make a post-mortem report: the 1926 Act, s.22, *post*, at p. 115. Alternatively, at the inquest the coroner may summon the deceased's registered medical practitioner, or another legally qualified medical practitioner in actual practice in or near where the death happened, to give evidence and direct him to make a post-mortem examination of the deceased: the Coroners Act 1887, s.21, *post* at p. 89.

    (*b*) Section 21 of the Coroners Act 1887 empowers a jury in certain circumstances to require the coroner to direct a post-mortem examination of the deceased.

[11] Coroners (Amendment) Act 1926, s.22, *post,* at p. 115. "Legally qualified medical practitioner": for definition see the Medical Act 1956, s.52(1).

RULE (The Coroners Rules 1984)	FORM (The Coroners Rules 1984, Schedule 4)

(2) The provisions relating to preservation of material and reporting restrictions in post-mortem examinations are applied to special examinations by rules 12 and 13. **12, 13**

9. After the outcome of the post-mortem (and special examination, if any) the coroner may carry out his own additional research *e.g.* checking records of operations or anaesthetics which might be relevant to the cause of death.[12]

10. If death natural, the coroner completes Pink Form "B"[13] and notifies the registrar of deaths that he does not intend to hold an inquest.

11. Registrar registers the cause of death recorded on Pink Form "B" by the coroner, who will have taken it from that certified by the pathologist on the post-mortem report.

12. Coroner decides to hold an inquest

The coroner notifies the date, hour and place of the inquest to:— **19**   **13**

(1) the spouse or a near relative or personal representative of the deceased whose name and address are known to the coroner; and

(2) (*a*) any other person, who, in the opinion of the coroner is within rule 20(2); and

(*b*) has asked the coroner to notify him of the aforesaid particulars of the inquest; and

(*c*) has supplied the coroner with his telephone number or address for the purpose of so notifying him.

---

[12] If the next of kin of the deceased wishes to have a second (private) post-mortem, this requires the coroner's consent. The coroner's pathologist should be informed and will normally attend such an examination.

[13] The Pink Form (specimen Form in Appendix, *post,* p. 29) comprises Parts A and B and is issued by the General Register Office for the purposes described in the Registration of Births, Deaths and Marriages Regulations 1968 (S.I. 1968 No. 2049).

	RULE (The Coroners Rules 1984)	FORM (The Coroners Rules 1984, Schedule 4)
13. The coroner is required to give reasonable notice of the date, hour and place of the inquest to any person whose conduct is likely to be called in question.[13a]	24, 25	
14. Coroner summons jury, if appropriate.[14]	44–53	3–5
15. Coroner summons witnesses.[14a]		8

INQUEST PROCEDURE

16. Preliminary inquest

(1) A preliminary hearing may precede the full inquest.[15] Evidence of the identity of the body and the pathologist's evidence may be given.

The Body:

The coroner may retain the body until the inquest is completed.[16]		
Alternatively, the coroner may release the body if he is satisfied that it is not required for further examination.		
It is not clear that he can be compelled to retain a body if he has decided to release it.		
The coroner can issue a burial order at any time after he has decided to hold an inquest.	14	21

[13a] Where a person whose conduct is likely to be called in question is in custody, the coroner should inform him through the governor of the prison unless the inquest is to be opened formally and adjourned immediately: Home Office Consolidated (Non-Industrial) Circular, No. 68/55.

[14] The Coroners (Amendment) Act 1926, s.13(2), *post,* at p. 108 lists circumstances in which a jury should be summoned.

[14a] If a person who is in custody is required by the coroner to attend, the coroner should apply to the Home Secretary for his production in court under the Prison Act, 1952, s.22(2)(*a*). Alternatively, he may apply to a High Court judge asking for the person to be produced: Criminal Procedure Act 1853.

[15] The Coroners (Amendment) Act 1926, s.13(4): "Where an inquest or any part of an inquest is held without a jury, anything done at the inquest, or at that part of the inquest, by or before the coroner alone shall be as validly done as if it had been done by or before the coroner and a jury."

[16] *R.* v. *Bristol Coroner, ex p. Kerr* [1974] Q.B. 652; [1974] 2 All E.R. 719, distinguished in *Re Aristos Constantinou, dec'd.,* Hornsey Coroners Court, January 10, 1985 (unreported). *Cf. Williams* v. *Williams* [1881] 20 Ch. 659: "Accordingly the law in this country is clear, that after the death of a man, his executors have a right to the custody and possession of his body (although they have no property in it) until it is properly buried," *per* Kay J. at p. 665.

	RULE (The Coroners Rules 1984)	FORM (The Coroners Rules 1984, Schedule 4)
A Cremation Certificate "E" can be issued at any time after the post-mortem examination has been completed or after the coroner has decided to hold an inquest provided the coroner is satisfied that the body is not required for further examination.[17]		
It is unusual at a preliminary hearing for a jury and legal representatives to be present. Legal aid is not available for inquests.		
(2) The inquest may be adjourned:[17a]		
To enable further inquiries to be made;		
To summon a jury and/or witnesses;		
At the request of a properly interested person;		
Where the death may have been caused by a notifiable disease or accident and the inspector or representative of the enforcing authority, etc. is absent;	23	
Where a person whose conduct is likely to be called in question is absent;	25	
Where the chief officer of police so requests on the ground that some person may be charged with murder, manslaughter, infanticide or causing death by reckless or dangerous driving or aiding, abetting, counselling or procuring suicide;	26	
Where the D.P.P. so requests on the ground that a person may be charged with an offence committed in circumstances connected with the death of the deceased, not being an offence within rule 26(3);	27	
In certain other cases.[18]	28	
A coroner has a general authority under his common law powers to adjourn an inquest for any		

[17] See n. 27, *post.*

[17a] An inquest should not be adjourned *sine die* but rather to a specific date unless there is express or implied statutory authority to the contrary. An inquest which is adjourned to a specific date but not resumed until a later day may be quashed on the ground that the inquest ended when the adjourned inquest was not resumed: *R.* v. *Payn* (1864) 34 L.J.Q.B. 59; *R.* v. *Coroner for Margate* (1865) 10 Cox C.C. 64.

[18] See (S.I. 1984 No. 552), r. 32, *post* for the effect of institution of criminal proceedings other than for homicide.

15

	RULE (The Coroners Rules 1984)	FORM (The Coroners Rules 1984, Schedule 4)
reasonable cause if he thinks fit (see Jervis, 9th ed. at p. 153). If the inquest is adjourned **then**:		
(3) (a) If the reason for the adjournment is listed in the Coroners (Amendment) Act 1926, s.20(1), the coroner furnishes a certificate to the registrar of deaths within five days;	29	
(b) If s.20(4) of the 1926 Act does not apply the coroner shall, on application, supply a properly interested person with an interim certificate of the fact of death. This enables the next of kin of the deceased to proceed with matters relating to, *e.g.* probate and social security benefits in the absence of a death certificate issued by a registrar;	30	14
(c) If adjournment was due to criminal proceedings which are then concluded, the coroner furnishes a certificate to the registrar of deaths.[19] Where such proceedings related to homicide the inquest is rarely resumed;[20]	31	
(d) In cases of homicide the coroner notifies the Crown Court officer of adjournment.	35	
and:		
(4) The coroner notifies persons as to (non) resumption of, and alteration of arrangements for, adjourned inquest;	33	15–18
If inquest adjourned pursuant to rule 23 the coroner gives such inspector or representative at least four days notice of the date, hour and place of holding of the adjourned inquest.	23	
(5) If the inquest is not resumed by the same coroner (or deputy or assistant deputy coroner) the original inquest becomes a nullity.[20a]		

[19] See, *ibid.* r. 31, *post*, at p. 50 for appropriate time limits.
[20] Coroners (Amendment) Act 1926, s.20(5), (7) and (8).
[20a] See Coroners (Amendment) Act 1926, s.14, now repealed by the Coroners Act 1980, s.1 and Sched. 1.

	RULE (The Coroners Rules 1984)	FORM (The Coroners Rules 1984, Schedule 4)

17. Full inquest

(1) Coroner opens inquest formally.[21] The ambit of inquiry is: who the deceased was, and how, when and where he came by his death.

(2) Submissions may be made, *e.g.* about the jury, concerning the disposal of the body, etc.

(3) In jury case, jury sworn in.[22]

(4) Coroner hears evidence of the identity of the body. Such evidence may already have been heard at the preliminary hearing.[23]

(5) View of locus, if coroner deems necessary.[23a]

(6) If the case is complex the coroner may outline the facts to the jury.

(7) Coroner swears in the witnesses. The court is inquisitorial and so the coroner examines each witness, taking a note of the evidence.

	RULE	FORM
(1)	16	
	36	
(3)		7
(7)		9
	39	

  (*a*) *Sequence of witnesses:*
    In order to assist the jury, the coroner will generally call the evidence in chronological order. Accordingly, unless the death was in police custody or resulted from an injury caused by a police officer in the purported execution of his duty, the police witnesses will usually give evidence towards the end of proceedings.
    Medical evidence may be given out of order, A G.P.'s evidence should generally precede the pathologist's evidence.

---

[21] r. 17: "Every inquest shall be held in public: Provided that the coroner may direct that the public be excluded from an inquest or any part of an inquest if he considers that it would be in the interest of national security so to do." See r. 18, *post* for days on which inquests should not be held.

[22] Coroners Act 1887, s.3(3): the jury must number at least seven.

[23] See n.15, *supra.*

[23a] If the jury view the locus, they must be sworn in beforehand. They should be placed in the care of the coroner's officer who should not discuss the inquest with them during the view. The jury must be kept separate from witnesses. The coroner has a discretion whether to permit interested persons or their legal representatives to be present at such a view: see *R.* v. *Divine, ex p. Walton* [1930] 2 K.B. 29.

	RULE (The Coroners Rules 1984)	FORM (The Coroners Rules 1984, Schedule 4)
A person whose conduct is likely to be called in question is entitled to know what is alleged against him. Accordingly, such persons will normally give evidence last.		
Properly interested persons or their legal representatives may examine each witness after the coroner. Rule 20, *post* lists the persons thus entitled.	20	

(b) Order of examination:

| Unless the coroner otherwise determines, a witness shall be examined first by the coroner and, if the witness is represented at the inquest, lastly by his or her representative.[23b] | 21 | |

(c) Scope of examination:

The proceedings should be confined to establishing identification, manner and cause of death.	36	
The coroner shall disallow any question which in his opinion is not relevant or is otherwise not a proper question.		
No witness shall be obliged to answer any question tending to incriminate himself. Where it appears to the coroner that a witness has been asked such a question, the coroner shall inform the witness that he may refuse to answer.[23c]	22	
It is permissable to put to a witness that he has made a previous inconsistent statement provided that it is done in accordance with the Criminal Procedure Act 1865, sections 3, 4 and 5 and the Civil Evidence Act 1968.		

[23b] The rules applicable to other Courts regarding the competence of witnesses to give evidence apply to a coroners' court. With regard to admissability of confessions the usual rules as to voluntariness apply also to coroners' proceedings: *R.* v. *Thompson* [1893] 2 Q.B. 12; *R.* v. *Unsworth* (1910) 6 Cr. App. R. 1.

[23c] See general note to r. 22, 1984 Rules, *post*, at p. 46, for the procedure when the privilege is claimed.

RULE (The Coroners Rules 1984)	FORM (The Coroners Rules 1984, Schedule 4)

(*d*) *Admissible evidence:*

Although the normal rules of evidence are followed in general at inquests, the strict rules of evidence of a criminal court do not apply to the Coroner's Court. Hearsay evidence is sometimes the only evidence available and may be admitted at the coroner's discretion.

(*e*) *Documentary evidence:*

Rule 37 provides that, "(1) Subject to the provisions of paragraphs (2) to (4), the coroner may admit at an inquest documentary evidence relevant to the purposes of the inquest from any living person which in his opinion is unlikely to be disputed, unless a person who in the opinion of the coroner is within rule 20(2) objects to the documentary evidence being admitted. **37**

(2) Documentary evidence so objected to may be admitted if in the opinion of the coroner the maker of the document is unable to give oral evidence within a reasonable period.

(3) Subject to paragraph (4), before admitting such documentary evidence the coroner shall at the beginning of the inquest announce publicly—

(a) that the documentary evidence may be admitted, and
(b) (i) the full name of the maker of the document to be admitted in evidence, and
(ii) a brief account of such document, and
(c) that any person who in the opinion of the coroner is within rule 20(2) may object to the admission of any such documentary evidence, and
(d) that any person who in the opinion of the coroner is within rule 20(2) is entitled to see

	RULE (The Coroners Rules 1984)	FORM (The Coroners Rules 1984, Schedule 4)

a copy of any such documentary evidence if he so wishes.

(4) If during the course of an inquest it appears that there is available at the inquest documentary evidence which in the opinion of the coroner is relevant to the purposes of the inquest but the maker of the document is not present and in the opinion of the coroner the content of the documentary evidence is unlikely to be disputed, the coroner shall at the earliest opportunity during the course of the inquest comply with the provisions of paragraph (3).

(5) A coroner may admit as evidence at an inquest any document made by a deceased person if he is of the opinion that the contents of the document are relevant to the purposes of the inquest.

(6) Any documentary evidence admitted under this rule shall, unless the coroner otherwise directs, be read aloud at the inquest."

There is no provision for taking unsworn evidence from children of tender years. Evidence of an interview by a woman police officer with the child may be given in such cases".[23d]

(f) Exhibits:

All exhibits should be marked with consecutive numbers and each number should be preceded by the letter "C." — 38

[23d] The position regarding unsworn evidence is not entirely clear. The Coroners Act 1887, s.4(1), *post*, at p. 82, requires all evidence to be given on oath. Nevertheless, it has been held that an inquisition will not be quashed solely on the ground that unsworn evidence was received: *R.* v. *Ingham* (1864) 5 B. & S. 257; and see *R.* v. *Staffordshire Coroner* (1864) 10 L.T. 650 and *R.* v. *Divine* [1930] 2 K.B. 29.

	RULE (The Coroners Rules 1984)	FORM (The Coroners Rules 1984, Schedule 4)
(8) No final speeches are permitted, nor may any person address the coroner or the jury as to the facts.[23e]	40	
(9) JURY-INQUEST		
(a) "In a jury inquest the coroner shall sum up the evidence to the jury and direct them as to the law before they consider their verdict and shall draw their attention to rules 36(2) and 42."	41	
(b) The jury retire to consider their verdict. A majority verdict may be accepted by the coroner but where more than two jurors disagree with the majority the coroner may discharge the jury and issue a warrant for summoning another jury. The old proceedings become a nullity and a new inquest is held.[24]		
(c) The jury deliver their verdict.[24a] No verdict shall be framed in such a way as to appear to determine any question of criminal on the part of a named person, or civil liability.	42	
(9A) NON-JURY-INQUEST		
The coroner announces his verdict.		
(10) After the verdict has been returned the coroner has a discretion to make an announcement and report of the type specified in Rule 43:	43	
"A coroner who believes that action should be taken to prevent the recurrence of fatalities		

[23e] A properly interested person or his representative may address the coroner as to the law.
[24] Coroners (Amendment) Act 1926, s.15(2).
[24a] It is improper for the coroner or anyone else to communicate with the jury or be present with them in the jury room while they are considering their verdict. If the jury wish to ask a question during their deliberations it must be done in open court: *R.* v. *Wood, ex p. Anderson* [1928] 1 K.B. 302; and see *R.* v. *Divine, ex p. Walton* [1930] 2 K.B. 29 and *R.* v. *Reynolds* [1945] K.B. 20.

The coroner is obliged to accept the jury's verdict, however perverse, if they persist in it after suitable explanation: *Smith's Case* (1696) Comb. 386. See further, commentary on r. 42, *post,* at p. 55, and commentary on 1984 Rules, Schedule 4, Form 22, *post,* at p. 72.

21

	RULE (The Coroners Rules 1984)	FORM (The Coroners Rules 1984, Schedule 4)

similar to that in respect of which the inquest is being held may announce at the inquest that he is reporting the matter in writing to the person or authority who may have power to take such action and he may report the matter accordingly."

(11) The inquisition is drawn up by the coroner and signed by him and the jury, if any.[25]

POST-INQUEST PROCEDURE

18. The coroner sends to the Registrar of Deaths the details required to be registered by the Births and Deaths Registration Act 1953 and such other certificates as are required by section 23(1) of the 1953 Act or section 20(5) and (7) of the 1926 Act as amended.

19. The registrar registers the death. If the death has already been registered, the details in the certificate are added to the entry in the register.

20. The coroner issues:

(1) a burial order, if he has not already done so[26]; **14**

or (2) a Cremation Certificate "E," if he has not already done so[27];

or (3) on application, permission for the body to be removed out of England and Wales.[28]

21. A coroner shall, on application by a properly **57** interested person and on payment of the prescribed fee (if any) supply to that person a copy of any post-mortem or special examination report, or of any notes of

[25] Coroners Act 1887, s.18(1).

[26] r. 14 states that a burial order can be issued at any time after the coroner has decided to hold an inquest. Note that a coroner cannot issue a burial order where he proposes to dispose of the case by post-mortem examination without an inquest, *i.e.* under the Coroners (Amendment) Act 1926, s.21, *post*, at p. 114.

[27] Cremation Regulations 1930 (S.R. & O. 1930 No. 1016) as amended by Cremation Regulations 1965 (S.I. 1965 No. 1146). A Cremation Certificate "E" can be issued at any time after the post-mortem examination has been completed or after the coroner has decided to hold an inquest provided the coroner is satisfied that the body is not required for further examination.

[28] Removal of Bodies Regulations (S.I. 1954 No. 448), reg 6.

evidence, or of any document put in evidence at the inquest.

22. Appeal

(1) *Coroners Act 1887, s.6*

(Application to have inquest held or inquisition quashed).

Grounds

"**6.** —(1) Where Her Majesty's High Court of Justice, upon application made by or under the authority of the Attorney General, is satisfied either—

(*a*) that a coroner refuses or neglects to hold an inquest which ought to be held; or

(*b*) where an inquest has been held by a coroner that by reason of fraud, rejection of evidence, irregularity of proceedings, insufficiency of inquiry, or otherwise, it is necessary or desirable, in the interests of justice, that another inquest should be held, the court may order an inquest to be held touching the said death, and may, if the court think it just, order the said coroner to pay such costs of and incidental to the application as to the court may seem just, and where an inquest has been already held may quash the inquisition on that inquest."[29]

Procedure

An application may be made by originating motion to the High Court. Such application may be by the Attorney General or under his statutory authority by an interested person.[30] The leave of the court is required[31] and, where an inquest has been held, the Court may quash the inquisition and order a fresh inquest to be held.[32]

(2) *R.S.C. Order 53*

(Application for judicial review).[33]

---

[29] Coroners Act 1887, s.6.

[30] "Interested person": includes the coroner, *Re an Application by the coroner for the West Derby Division of Lancashire* [1954] Crim.L.R. 373, also the Crown, *Re Culley* (1833) 5 B. & Ad. 230.

An interested person seeking relief under the 1887 Act, s.6, should send a memorial to the Attorney General together with a statutory declaration to verify it. It is usual to file an affidavit by the coroner verifying a copy of the inquisition or explaining its absence.

[31] *R. v. South London Coroner, ex p. Thompson and Others, The Times,* July 9, 1982, *per* Comyn J.

[32] Coroners Act 1887, ss.6, 35.

[33] There is also a common law power by order of *certiorari* addressed to a coroner, to apply to the Q.B.D. to have an inquisition quashed.

Grounds

The usual grounds for judicial review[34] including a jurisdictional error of law by the coroner.[35]

Procedure

An application may be made *ex parte* by originating motion to a judge in open court[36] to have the inquisition quashed or the verdict amended.[37] The applicant must, in the court's opinion, have a "sufficient interest in the matter to which the application relates."[38] Leave of the Court is required.[39] The coroner will normally respond by affidavit.[40]

---

[34] Lord Reid listed some of these grounds in *Anisminic* v. *Foreign Compensation Commission* [1969] 2 A.C. 147, H.C. at 171 paras. B–D:

> "It has sometimes been said that it is only where a tribunal acts without jurisdiction that its decision is a nullity. But in such cases the word "jurisdiction" has been used in a very wide sense, and I have come to the conclusion that it is better not to use the term except in the narrow and original sense of the tribunal being entitled to enter on the inquiry in question. But there are many cases where, although the tribunal had jurisdiction to enter on the inquiry, it has done or failed to do something in the course of the inquiry which is of such a nature that its decision is a nullity. It may have given its decision in bad faith. It may have made a decision which it had no power to make. It may have failed in the course of the inquiry to comply with the requirements of natural justice. It may in perfect good faith have misconstrued the provisions giving it power to act so that it failed to deal with the question remitted to it and decided some question which was not remitted to it. It may have refused to take into account something which it was required to take into account. Or it may have based its decision on some matter which, under the provisions setting it up, it had no right to take into account. I do not intend this list to be exhaustive."

See now Lord Diplock's restatement of the grounds in *Council of Civil Service Unions* v. *Minister for the Civil Service* [1984] 3 W.L.R. 1174; [1984] 3 All E.R. 935 at p. 949. See also *R.* v. *Divine, ex p. Walton* [1930] 2 K.B. 29: the High Court will not quash a coroner's verdict where the irregularity is slight or unimportant but if the inquest has been so conducted that there is a real risk that justice has not been done, the inquisition will be quashed. *Re Davis* [1967] 2 W.L.R. 1089; [1967] 1 All E.R. 688, C.A.: a coroner's verdict cannot be quashed on certiorari unless a different verdict will probably result. *R.* v. *Cardiff Coroner, ex p. Thomas* [1970] 3 All E.R. 469, D.C.: where the applicant for an order for certiorari had made out a case for the inquisition to be quashed, new affidavit evidence adduced by the coroner after the inquest was not a reason to refuse the order.

[35] *R.* v. *Greater Manchester Coroner, ex p. Tal* [1984] 3 All E.R. 240, D.C. It is no longer a requirement of judicial review in coroners' cases that an error of law which is sought to be reviewed appears on the face of the record *cf. R.* v. *Surrey Coroner, ex p. Campbell* [1982] Q.B. 661.

[36] R.S.C. Ord. 53, r.5.

[37] See *R.* v. *H.M. Coroner for the County of London, ex p. Rubenstein, The Times,* February 24, 1982.

[38] R.S.C. Ord. 53, r.3(5). See 9 *Halsbury's Laws* (4th ed.), para. 1144 for persons aggrieved by an inquisition and who therefore have the locus to apply for judicial review and see *R.* v. *I.R.C., ex p. National Federation of Self Employed and Small Businesses Ltd.* [1982] A.C. 617, for discussion of who has a sufficient interest.

[39] R.S.C. Ord. 53, r.3(1).

[40] See *R.* v. *Huntbach, ex p. Lockley* [1944] 2 All E.R. 453, D.C. for the type of detail required in the affidavit.

24

23. Use of evidence adduced at an inquest in subsequent proceedings

(1) *Coroner's Notes of Evidence in Subsequent Civil Proceedings*

In civil proceedings neither the inquisition nor the record of evidence given in a coroner's court is admissible in evidence, but they may be used for the purposes of cross examination.[41] Before they are so used, they should be properly proved. Strictly, this would require the coroner to come to the trial but, as an alternative, an order may be made as follows:

> "That a copy of the notes of evidence taken at the coroner's inquest upon the deceased (duly certified by the coroner or his officer or agreed between the parties) be admissible at the trial for the same purposes and to the same extent as the contents of the original would have been if duly proved by the coroner (or the person who took down the same) without calling the coroner (or such person) and without proving the original or copy."[42]

(2) *Coroner's Notes of Evidence in Subsequent Criminal Proceedings*

It is no longer the practice for coroners to take depositions and it is misleading to use that term nowadays in the context of inquest evidence.

Before 1977 the coroner took depositions only in cases of murder, manslaughter and infanticide, causing death by dangerous or reckless driving and aiding, abetting, counselling or procuring a suicide. The Coroners Act 1887, section 5(3) provided for these depositions to be furnished to the court of trial if the coroner committed a person for trial on any of these charges. Section 5(3) of the 1887 Act was repealed by the Criminal Law Act 1977, s.65(5) and Schedule 13. That Act abolished the coroner's criminal jurisdiction altogether. Now, if the evidence points to homicide by a named person, the coroner must adjourn the inquest under rule 28 of the 1984 Rules and refer the papers to the D.P.P.

Nevertheless, there remain instances where a criminal prosecution, *e.g.* for careless driving, may follow an inquest. In such cases the coroner will normally furnish the trial court with a copy of the notes of inquest evidence, if requested to do so. By virtue of the Criminal Procedure Act 1865, sections 4 and 5, such notes may be used to cross-examine a witness on the basis that he has previously given evidence inconsistent with his testimony in the trial court. (See Archbold, *Pleading, Evidence and Practice in Criminal Cases (41st ed., 1982), paras. 4-318 et seq.* and *see para. 4-321* as to whether the previous testimony becomes evidence in the trial).

The facts found in an inquisition, or the opinion of the jury expressed in the verdict, cannot be used in subsequent proceedings (civil or criminal) as evidence that those facts or opinions were necessarily true: *Barnett* v. *Cohen* [1921] 2 K.B. 461; *Bird* v. *Keep* [1918] 2 K.B. 699.

---

[41] *Per* Lord Dunedin in *Calmenson* v. *Merchants' Warehousing Co.* [1921] W.N. 59, (1921) 90 L.J.P.C. 134; *Barnett* v. *Cohen* [1921] 2 K.B. 461; *Bird* v. *Keep* [1918] 2 K.B. 692, C.A., at p. 699.

[42] R.S.C. Ord. 25, r. 3, see *Supreme Court Practice* 1985, para. 25/3/3, at p. 425.

APPENDIX TO PROCEDURE

SPECIMEN PINK FORM "A" AND "B"

NOTIFICATION TO THE REGISTRAR BY THE CORONER THAT HE DOES NOT INTEND TO HOLD AN INQUEST

NOTIFICATION TO THE REGISTRAR BY THE CORONER
that he does not consider it necessary to hold an Inquest

For completion by coroner	If a histological or bacteriological examination is to be made, please initial ➞		For completion by registrar	Entry No.

A.

For use where **NO POST-MORTEM** has been held under Section 21 of the Coroners (Amendment) Act, 1926

PARTICULARS OF DECEASED PERSON—Name and surname.......................................

Age...................Date and place of death...

Cause of death:

*

    The circumstances connected with the death of the above person have been reported to me and I do not consider it necessary to hold an inquest.

Signature.................................. H.M. Coroner for.......................... Date.............

To:..Registrar of births and deaths.
Where this notification relates to a still-born child this should be stated here.

B.

For use where a **POST-MORTEM** has been held under Section 21 of the Coroners (Amendment) Act, 1926

PARTICULARS OF DECEASED PERSON—Name and surname.................................

Age...................Date and place of death...

*

I hereby certify that a post-mortem examination of the body of the

above person was made by.................................
and his report disclosed that the cause of death was:

*I have given a Certificate E

for cremation dated...to

(name) ....of

(address) ....

*Delete words in italics if not applicable

and I am satisfied that an inquest is unnecessary.

Signature.................................. H.M. Coroner for.......................... Date.............

To:..Registrar of births and deaths
Where this notification relates to a still-born child this should be stated here.

INSTRUCTIONS TO REGISTRAR

This death must be registered in the presence of an ordinary informant and spaces 1-7 should be completed in accordance with the information given by the informant and not copied from this form.

    If **A is filled up** and the deceased was attended during his last illness by a registered medical practitioner, the cause of death must be entered from the certificate issued by him and not from this form.

    If **B is filled up** the cause of death must be entered from this form as in Example No. 28 or 32 in Appendix O of the Handbook

    If **B relates to** a still-birth then the pathologist's certificate should be sent with this form, if not, you must request the Coroner to forward it.   **Form 100**

MODEL MEDICAL CERTIFICATE OF CAUSE OF DEATH

30

Complete where applicable

A	B
I have reported this death to the Coroner for further action.	I may be in a position later to give, on application by the Registrar General, additional information as to the cause of death for the purpose of more precise statistical classification.
Initials of certifying medical practitioner.	Initials of certifying medical practitioner.

The Coroner needs to consider all cases where:

The death might have been due to or contributed to by a violent or unnatural cause (including an accident);

or the cause of death cannot be identified;

or the death might have been due to or contributed to by drugs, medicine, abortion or poison;

or there is reason to believe that the death occurred during an operation or under or prior to complete recovery from an anaesthetic or arising subsequently out of an incident during an operation or an anaesthetic;

or the death might have been due to or contributed to by the employment followed at some time by the deceased.

LIST OF SOME OF THE CATEGORIES OF DEATH WHICH MAY BE OF INDUSTRIAL ORIGIN

MALIGNANT DISEASES — Causes include:

(a) Skin — radiation and sunlight, pitch or tar, mineral oils
(b) Nasal — wood or leather work, nickel
(c) Lung — asbestos, nickel, radiation
(d) Pleura — asbestos
(e) Urinary Tract — benzidine, dyestuff, chemicals in rubbers
(f) Liver — PVC manufacture
(g) Bone — radiation
(h) Lymphatics and haematopoietic — radiation, benzene

POISONING

(a) Metals — e.g. arsenics, cadmium, lead
(b) Chemicals — e.g. chlorine, benzene
(c) Solvents — e.g. trichlorethylene

INFECTIOUS DISEASES — Causes include:

(a) Anthrax — imported bone, bonemeal, hide or fur
(b) Brucellosis — farming or veterinary
(c) Tuberculosis — contact at work
(d) Leptospirosis — farming, sewer or underground workers
(e) Tetanus — farming or gardening
(f) Rabies — animal handling
(g) Viral hepatitis — contact at work

BRONCHIAL ASTHMA AND PNEUMONITIS

(a) Occupational asthma — sensitising agent at work
(b) Allergic Alveolitis — farming

PNEUMOCONIOSIS — mining and quarrying, pottery, asbestos

NOTE:—The Practitioner, on signing the certificate, should complete, sign and date the Notice to the Informant, which should be detached and handed to the Informant. The Practitioner should then, without delay, deliver the certificate itself to the Registrar of Births and Deaths for the sub-district in which the death occurred. Envelopes for enclosing the certificates are supplied by the Registrar.

PERSONS QUALIFIED AND LIABLE TO ACT AS INFORMANTS

The following persons are designated by the Births and Deaths Registration Act 1953 as qualified to give information concerning a death:—

DEATHS IN HOUSES AND PUBLIC INSTITUTIONS

(1) A relative of the deceased, present at the death.
(2) A relative of the deceased, in attendance during the last illness.
(3) A relative of the deceased, residing or being in the sub-district where the death occurred.
(4) A person present at the death.
(5) The occupier* if he knew of the happening of the death.
(6) Any inmate if he knew of the happening of the death.
(7) The person causing the disposal of the body.

DEATHS NOT IN HOUSES OR DEAD BODIES FOUND

(1) Any relative of the deceased having knowledge of any of the particulars required to be registered.
(2) Any person present at the death.
(3) Any person who found the body.
(4) Any person in charge of the body.
(5) The person causing the disposal of the body.

*"Occupier" in relation to a public institution includes the governor, keeper, master, matron, superintendent, or other chief resident officer.

The design of this form is Crown copyright and is reproduced with the permission of the Controller of Her Majesty's Stationery Office.

THE CORONERS RULES 1984

THE CORONERS RULES 1984

(S.I. 1984 No. 552)

Made - - - - -	*9th April* 1984
Came into Operation	1*st July* 1984

ARRANGEMENT OF RULES

PART I

General

PART II

Availability of Coroner

PART III

Post-Mortem Examinations

PART IV

Special Examinations

Part V

Burial Orders

Part VI

Inquests

PART VII

Summoning of Jurors and Excusal from Jury Service

PART VIII

Records, Documents, Exhibits and Forms

SCHEDULES

Schedule 1: Revocations.

Schedule 2: Post-Mortem Examination Report.

Schedule 3: Register of Deaths Reported to the Coroner.

Schedule 4: Forms.

The Lord Chancellor, in exercise of the powers conferred on him by sections 26 and 27 of the Coroners (Amendment) Act 1926 and with the concurrence of the Secretary of State, hereby makes the following Rules:—

COMMENTARY

Section 26 was amended by Coroners' Juries Act 1983, s.2.

RULE 1

Citation and commencement

1. These Rules may be cited as the Coroners Rules 1984 and shall come into operation on 1st July 1984.

RULE 2

Interpretation

2. (1) In these Rules, unless the context otherwise requires—
"the Act of 1887" means the Coroners Act 1887;
"the Act of 1926" means the Coroners (Amendment) Act 1926;
"appropriate officer" has the same meaning as it has in section 3A of the Act of 1887;
"chief officer of police" means the chief officer of police for the area in which the coroner's jurisdiction is comprised;
"coroner" includes a deputy and assistant deputy coroner;
"deceased" means the person upon whose body a post-mortem examination is made or touching whose death an inquest is held or the person whose death is reported to the coroner, as the case may be;
"enforcing authority" has the same meaning as it has in section 18(7) of the Health and Safety at Work etc. Act 1974;
"hospital" means any institution for the reception and treatment of persons suffering from illness or mental disorder, any maternity home, and any institution for the reception and treatment of persons during convalescence;
"industrial disease" means a disease prescribed under section 76 of the Social Security Act 1975;
"inquest" means an inquest for the purpose of inquiring into the death of a person;
"legal proceedings" includes proceedings for the purpose of obtaining any benefit or other payments under the provisions of the Social Security Act 1975 relating to industrial injuries or under section 5 of the Industrial Injuries and Diseases (Old Cases) Act 1975:
"pneumoconiosis medical board" and "pneumoconiosis medical panel" have the same meaning as they have in the Social Security (Industrial Injuries) (Prescribed Diseases) Regulations 1980;
"post-mortem examination" means a post-mortem examination which a legally qualified medical practitioner is directed or requested by a coroner to make under section 21 of the Act of 1887 or under section 21(1) or 22(1) of the Act of 1926;
"registrar" means a registrar of births and deaths;

"the Registration Acts" has the same meaning as it has in the Act of 1887;
"special examination" has the same meaning as it has in section 22(1) of
the Act of 1926.

(2) In these Rules any reference to a Rule or Schedule shall be construed
as a reference to a Rule contained in these Rules, or, as the case may be, to a
Schedule thereto; and any reference in a Rule to a paragraph shall be
construed as a reference to a paragraph of that Rule.

COMMENTARY ON RULE 2

"appropriate officer." Section 3A of the Act of 1887 was inserted by
Coroners' Juries Act 1983, s.1.

RULE 3

Revocations and application

3. (1) Subject to paragraph (2), the Rules specified in Schedule 1 are
hereby revoked.

(2) These Rules shall not have effect in relation to any inquest begun
before 1st July 1984 or to any post-mortem examination which, before that
day, a coroner has directed or requested a medical practitioner to make; and,
accordingly, the Rules revoked by paragraph (1) shall continue to have
effect in relation to any such inquest or post-mortem examination.

RULE 4

Coroner to be available at all times

4. A coroner shall at all times hold himself ready to undertake, either by
himself or by his deputy or assistant deputy, any duties in connection with
inquests and post-mortem examinations.

RULE 5

Delay in making post-mortem to be avoided

5. Where a coroner directs or requests that a post-mortem examination
shall be made, it shall be made as soon after the death of the deceased as is
reasonably practicable.

COMMENTARY ON RULE 5

General Note

See definition of post-mortem examination in rule 2(1), *ante.* For standard form
Post-Mortem Examination Report, see Schedule 2, *post.*

RULE 6

Medical practitioner making post-mortem

6. (1) In considering what legally qualified medical practitioner shall be directed or requested by the coroner to make a post-mortem examination the coroner shall have regard to the following considerations:

(*a*) the post-mortem examination should be made, whenever practicable, by a pathologist with suitable qualifications and experience and having access to laboratory facilities;

(*b*) if the coroner is informed by the chief officer of police that a person may be charged with the murder, manslaughter or infanticide of the deceased, the coroner should consult the chief officer of police regarding the legally qualified medical practitioner who is to make the post-mortem examination;

(*c*) if the deceased died in a hospital, the coroner should not direct or request a pathologist on the staff of, or associated with, that hospital to make a post-mortem examination if

(i) that pathologist does not desire to make the examination, or

(ii) the conduct of any member of the hospital staff is likely to be called in question, or

(iii) any relative of the deceased asks the coroner that the examination be not made by such a pathologist,

unless the obtaining of another pathologist with suitable qualifications and experience would cause the examination to be unduly delayed;

(*d*) if the death of the deceased may have been caused by any of the diseases or injuries within paragraph (2), the coroner should not direct or request a legally qualified medical practitioner who is a member of a pneumoconiosis medical panel to make the post-mortem examination.

(2) The diseases and injuries within this paragraph are those in connection with which duties are from time to time imposed upon pneumoconiosis medical boards by Part III of the Social Security Act 1975 and any regulations made under that Act.

COMMENTARY ON RULE 6

General Note

"Legally qualified medical practitioner" in subsection (1): for definition see the Medical Act 1956, s.52(1).

For the appropriate Form directing medical practitioner to make post-mortem examination see Schedule 4, Form 10, *post.*

The provisions in rule 6(2) are new to the 1984 Rules, *cf.* S.I. 1953 No. 205, rule 3. This part of the rule was made necessary for the sake of greater precision in identifying the causes of death referred to in rule 6(1)(*d*). Rule 3(*d*) of the 1953 Rules (replaced by rule 6(1)(*d*) of the 1984 Rules) referred to the cause of death simply as "pneumoconiosis," a term which covers a number of specific diseases.

RULE 7

Coroner to notify persons of post-mortem to be made

7. (1) Where a coroner directs or requests a legally qualified medical practitioner to make a post-mortem examination, the coroner shall notify the persons and bodies set out in paragraph (2) of the date, hour and place at which the examination will be made, unless it is impracticable to notify any such persons or bodies or to do so would cause the examination to be unduly delayed.

(2) The persons and bodies to be notified by the coroner are as follows:
  (*a*) any relative of the deceased who has notified the coroner of his desire to attend, or be represented at, the post-mortem examination;
  (*b*) the deceased's regular medical attendant;
  (*c*) if the deceased died in a hospital, the hospital;
  (*d*) if the death of the deceased may have been caused by any of the diseases or injuries within Rule 6(2) (other than occupational asthma), the pneumoconiosis medical panel for the area;
  (*e*) if the death of the deceased may have been caused by any accident or disease notice of which is required by or under any enactment to be given
    (i) to an enforcing authority, the appropriate inspector appointed by, or representative of, that authority; or
    (ii) to an inspector appointed by an enforcing authority, that inspector;
  (*f*) any government department which has notified the coroner of its desire to be represented at the examination;
  (*g*) if the chief officer of police has notified the coroner of his desire to be represented at the examination, the chief officer of police.

(3) Any person or body mentioned in paragraph (2) shall be entitled to be represented at a post-mortem examination by a legally qualified medical practitioner, or if any such person is a legally qualified medical practitioner he shall be entitled to attend the examination in person; but the chief officer of police may be represented by a member of the police force of which he is chief officer.

(4) Nothing in the foregoing provisions of this Rule shall be deemed to limit the discretion of the coroner to notify any person of the date, hour and place at which a post-mortem examination will be made and to permit him to attend the examination.

General Note

The new subsection (*e*) expands the old rule 4(2)(*e*) (1953 Rules) which reads: "If the death of the deceased may have been caused by any accident or disease of which notice is required by the Factories Act 1937 to be given to an Inspector of Factories for the district." It was made necessary by the provisions of the Health and Safety at Work, etc., Act 1974. Inspectors appointed under that Act assumed the function of Factory Inspectors.

RULE 8

Persons attending post-mortem not to interfere

8. A person attending a post-mortem examination by virtue of paragraph (3) or (4) of Rule 7 shall not interfere with the performance of the examination.

RULE 9

Preservation of material

9. A person making a post-mortem examination shall make provision, so far as possible, for the preservation of material which in his opinion bears upon the cause of death for such period as the coroner thinks fit.

RULE 10

Report on post-mortem

10. (1) The person making a post-mortem examination shall report to the coroner in the form set out in Schedule 2 or in a form to the like effect.

(2) Unless authorised by the coroner, the person making a post-mortem examination shall not supply a copy of his report to any person other than the coroner.

RULE 11

Premises for post-mortems

11. (1) No post-mortem examination shall be made in a dwelling house or in licensed premises.

(2) Every post-mortem examination shall be made in premises which are adequately equipped for the purpose of the examination.

(3) Where a person dies in a hospital possessing premises so equipped, any post-mortem examination of the body of that person shall, with the consent of the hospital authority, be made in those premises unless the coroner otherwise decides.

(4) For the purpose of this Rule no premises shall be deemed to be adequately equipped for the purpose of post-mortem examinations unless they are supplied with running water, proper heating and lighting facilities, and containers for the storing and preservation of material.

RULE 12

Preservation of material

12. A person making a special examination shall make provision, so far as possible, for the preservation of the material submitted to him for examination for such period as the coroner thinks fit.

RULE 13

Report on special examination

13. Unless authorised by the coroner, the person making a special examination shall not supply a copy of his report to any person other than the coroner.

RULE 14

Issue of burial order

14. An order of a coroner authorising the burial of a body shall not be issued unless the coroner has held, or has decided to hold, an inquest touching the death.

COMMENTARY ON RULE 14

General Note

If a coroner holds or decides to hold an inquest then he may issue a burial order. It is unlawful to dispose of the body of a deceased person before a registrar's certificate or coroner's order has been delivered to the person disposing of the body: Births and Deaths Registration Act 1926 (c.48), s.1. A coroner cannot issue a burial order where he proposes to dispose of the case by post-mortem examination without an inquest, *i.e.* under the Coroners (Amendment) Act 1926, s.21, *post*, at page 114.

See note 16, *ante*, at page 14 for the coroner's common law right to retain the body.

RULE 15

Burial order where certificate for disposal of body issued

15. Where a coroner is satisfied that a certificate for the disposal of a body has been issued by a registrar, the coroner shall not issue an order authorising the burial of that body unless the certificate has been surrendered to him; and in such a case he shall on issuing the order transmit the certificate to the registrar and inform him of the issue of the order.

RULE 16

Formality

16. Every inquest shall be opened, adjourned and closed in a formal manner.

RULE 17

Inquest in public

17. Every inquest shall be held in public:

Provided that the coroner may direct that the public be excluded from an inquest or any part of an inquest if he considers that it would be in the interest of national security to do so.

COMMENTARY ON RULE 17

General Note

It is unlawful to take photographs or make sketches in, or in the vicinity of a coroner's court: see the Criminal Justice Act, 1925, s.41.

Contemporaneous reports of proceedings in the coroner's court, if fair and accurate, are absolutely privileged: *McCarey* v. *Associated Newspapers Ltd.* [1964] 1 W.L.R. 854, *per* Thompson, J.

RULE 18

Days on which inquest not to be held

18. An inquest shall not be held on Christmas Day, Good Friday, or a Bank Holiday unless the coroner thinks it requisite on grounds of urgency that an inquest should be held on such a day, and no inquest shall be held on a Sunday.

RULE 19

Coroner to notify persons of inquest arrangements

19. The coroner shall notify the date, hour and place of an inquest to

(*a*) the spouse or a near relative or personal representative of the deceased whose name and address are known to the coroner; and

44

(*b*) any other person who

  (i) in the opinion of the coroner is within Rule 20(2); and

  (ii) has asked the coroner to notify him of the aforesaid particulars of the inquest; and

  (iii) has supplied the coroner with a telephone number or address for the purpose of so notifying him.

COMMENTARY ON RULE 19

General Note

"Coroner to notify persons of inquest arrangements." The appropriate Form of Notice is set out in Schedule 4, Form 13, *post*, at page 69.

RULE 20

Entitlement to examine witnesses

20. (1) Without prejudice to any enactment with regard to the examination of witnesses at an inquest, any person who satisfies the coroner that he is within paragraph (2) shall be entitled to examine any witness at an inquest either in person or by counsel or solicitor:
Provided that

(*a*) the chief officer of police, unless interested otherwise than in that capacity, shall only be entitled to examine a witness by counsel or solicitor;

(*b*) the coroner shall disallow any question which in his opinion is not relevant or is otherwise not a proper question.

(2) Each of the following persons shall have the rights conferred by paragraph (1):

(*a*) a parent, child, spouse and any personal representative of the deceased;

(*b*) any beneficiary under a policy of insurance issued on the life of the deceased;

(*c*) the insurer who issued such a policy of insurance;

(*d*) any person whose act or omission or that of his agent or servant may in the opinion of the coroner have caused, or contributed to, the death of the deceased;

(*e*) any person appointed by a trade union to which the deceased at the time of his death belonged, if the death of the deceased may have been caused by an injury received in the course of his employment or by an industrial disease;

45

(*f*) an inspector appointed by, or a representative of, an enforcing authority, or any person appointed by a government department to attend the inquest;

(*g*) the chief officer of police;

(*h*) any other person who, in the opinion of the coroner, is a properly interested person.

COMMENTARY ON RULE 20

General Note

"any enactment with regard to the examination of witnesses at an inquest," in rule 20(1): see the Coroners Act 1887 (c.71), s.4(1).

"Solicitor" in rule 20(1) does not include managing clerk.

Forms

Summons to Witness, Schedule 4, Form 8, *post.* Witness Oath, Schedule 4, Form 9, *post.*

RULE 21

Examination of witnesses

21. Unless the coroner otherwise determines, a witness at an inquest shall be examined first by the coroner and, if the witness is represented at the inquest, lastly by his representative.

RULE 22

Self-incrimination

22. (1) No witness at an inquest shall be obliged to answer any question tending to incriminate himself.

(2) Where it appears to the coroner that a witness has been asked such a question, the coroner shall inform the witness that he may refuse to answer.

COMMENTARY ON RULE 22

General Note

"tending to incriminate", see Phipson on Evidence (13th ed., 1982), at page 314. A witness cannot refuse to go into the box on the ground that he might incriminate himself; he can only claim privilege after he has been sworn and the question put: *Wakley* v. *Cooke* (1849) 4 Ex. 511; *Boyle* v. *Wiseman* (1855) 10 Ex. 647.

It is for the witness or his representative to object. It is for the coroner to decide whether or not the witness is entitled to the privilege.

The privilege covers both giving oral evidence and producing documents: *Spokes* v. *Grosvenor Hotel* [1897] 2 Q.B. 124. Note that the evidence which a witness refuses to give may be proved in other ways, *e.g.* by another witness's testimony.

RULE 23

Adjournment where inspector or representative of enforcing authority etc. is not present

23. (1) Where a coroner holds an inquest touching the death of a person which may have been caused by an accident or disease notice of which is required to be given to an enforcing authority, the coroner shall adjourn the inquest unless an inspector appointed by, or a representative of, the enforcing authority is present to watch the proceedings and shall, at least four days before holding the adjourned inquest, give to such inspector or representative notice of the date, hour and place of holding the adjourned inquest.

(2) Where a coroner holds an inquest touching the death of a person which may have been caused by an accident or disease, notice of which is required to be given to an inspector appointed by an enforcing authority, the coroner shall adjourn the inquest unless the inspector or a representative of the inspector is present to watch the proceedings and shall, at least four days before holding the adjourned inquest, give to the inspector or representative notice of the date, hour and place of holding the adjourned inquest.

COMMENTARY ON RULE 23

General Note

The substance of rule 23, which was agreed with the Health and Safety Executive, interprets the provisions of Regulations made under the Health and Safety at Work, etc. Act 1974 (S.I. 1980 No. 804) in which the persons appointed either under the Act or by an enforcing authority had been somewhat changed in definition.

RULE 24

Notice to person whose conduct is likely to be called in question

24. Any person whose conduct is likely in the opinion of the coroner to be called in question at an inquest shall, if not duly summoned to give evidence at the inquest, be given reasonable notice of the date, hour and place at which the inquest will be held.

COMMENTARY ON RULE 24

General Note

See notes 13a and 14a, *ante*, at page 14.

RULE 25

Adjournment where person whose conduct is called in question is not present

25. If the conduct of any person is called in question at an inquest on grounds which the coroner thinks substantial and which relate to any matter referred to in Rule 36 and if that person is not present at the inquest and has not been duly summoned to attend or otherwise given notice of the holding of the inquest, the inquest shall be adjourned to enable him to be present, if he so desires.

RULE 26

Request by chief officer of police for adjournment

26. (1) If the chief officer of police requests a coroner to adjourn an inquest on the ground that a person may be charged with an offence within paragraph (3), the coroner shall adjourn the inquest for twenty-eight days or for such longer period as he may think fit.

(2) At any time before the date fixed for the holding of the adjourned inquest, the chief officer of police may ask the coroner for a further adjournment and the coroner may comply with his request.

(3) The offences within this paragraph are murder, manslaughter or infanticide of the deceased, an offence under section 1 of the Road Traffic Act 1972 committed by causing the death of the deceased and an offence under section 2(1) of the Suicide Act 1961 consisting of aiding, abetting, counselling or procuring the suicide of the deceased.

COMMENTARY ON RULE 26

General Note

"Adjourn an inquest" in rule 26(1). For adjournment see also the 1926 Act, s.20 and rules 32 and 33, *post.*

The reference to adjournment for 28 days at the request of the chief officer of police was inserted in the 1953 Rules by the Coroners (Amendment) Rules 1977 (S.I. 1977 No. 1881). It amended rule 22(1) of the 1953 Rules which provided for adjournment for a period of 14 days in the same circumstances.

RULE 27

Request by Director of Public Prosecutions for adjournment

27. (1) If the Director of Public Prosecutions requests a coroner to adjourn an inquest on the ground that a person may be charged with an offence (whether or not involving the death of a person other than the deceased) committed in circumstances connected with the death of the deceased, not being an offence within Rule 26(3), the coroner shall adjourn the inquest for twenty-eight days or for such longer period as he may think fit.

(2) At any time before the date fixed for the holding of the adjourned inquest, the Director of Public Prosecutions may ask the coroner for a further adjournment and the coroner may comply with his request.

COMMENTARY ON RULE 27

General Note

See also s.20(1)(*b*) of the 1926 Act, *post,* at page 112.

The provisions in rule 27(1) were inserted in the 1953 Rules by the Coroners (Amendment) Rules 1977 (S.I. 1977 No. 1881).

The provisions in rule 27(2) are new.

RULE 28

Coroner to adjourn in certain other cases

28. (1) If during the course of an inquest evidence is given from which it appears to the coroner that the death of the deceased is likely to be due to an offence within Rule 26(3) and that a person might be charged with such an offence, then the coroner, unless he has previously been notified by the Director of Public Prosecutions that adjournment is unnecessary, shall adjourn the inquest for fourteen days or for such longer period as he may think fit and send to the Director particulars of that evidence.

(2) At any time before the date fixed for the holding of the adjourned inquest, the Director of Public Prosecutions may ask the coroner for a further adjournment and the coroner may comply with his request.

COMMENTARY ON RULE 28

General Note

The provisions in rule 28(1) were inserted in the 1953 Rules by the Coroners (Amendment) Rules 1977 (S.I. 1977, No. 1881).

The provisions in rule 28(2) are new.

For adjournments generally see note 17a, *ante,* at page 15.

RULE 29

Coroner to furnish certificate after adjournment

29. A certificate under the hand of a coroner stating the particulars which under the Registration Acts are required to be registered concerning a death which he furnishes to a registrar of deaths under section 20(4)(a) of the Act of 1926 shall be furnished within five days from the date on which the inquest is adjourned.

COMMENTARY ON RULE 29

General Note

The Registration Acts currently in force are the Births and Deaths Registration Act 1926 and the Births and Deaths Registration Act 1953. The Rule is framed so that it automatically refers to the statutes currently in force at any time.

RULE 30

Coroner's interim certificate of the fact of death

30. When an inquest has been adjourned for any reason and section 20(4) of the Act of 1926 does not apply, the coroner shall on application supply to any person who, in the opinion of the coroner, is a properly interested person an interim certificate of the fact of death.

COMMENTARY ON RULE 30

General Note

Rule 30 is a new provision.

Forms

See Schedule 4, Form 14, *post*, at page 70.

RULE 31

Coroner to furnish certificate stating result of criminal proceedings

31. A certificate under the hand of a coroner stating the result of the relevant criminal proceedings which he furnishes to a registrar of deaths under section 20(5) or section 20(7) of the Act of 1926 shall be furnished within twenty-eight days from the date on which he is notified of the result of the proceedings under section 20(9) or section 20(10) of that Act or, if the person charged with an offence before a magistrates' court as mentioned in section 20(8) of that Act is not committed for trial to the Crown Court, within twenty-eight days from the date on which he is notified under the said section 20(8) of the result of the proceedings in the magistrates' court.

RULE 32

Effect of institution of criminal proceedings

32. Subject to section 20 of the Act of 1926, an inquest shall not be adjourned solely by reason of the institution of criminal proceedings arising out of the death of the deceased.

COMMENTARY ON RULE 32

General Note

"Pending the conclusion of an inquest the police should not prefer a lesser charge, or if it is preferred, it should not be heard or determined": *Re Beresford* [1952] 36 Cr. App. R.1, *obiter, per* Devlin.J.

RULE 33

Coroner to notify persons as to resumption of, and alteration of arrangements for, adjourned inquest

33. (1) If an inquest which has been adjourned in pursuance of section 20 of the Act of 1926 is not to be resumed, the coroner shall notify the persons within paragraph (4).

(2) If an inquest which has been adjourned as aforesaid is to be resumed, the coroner shall give reasonable notice of the date, hour and place at which the inquest will be resumed to the persons within paragraph (4).

(3) Where a coroner has fixed a date, hour and place for the holding of an inquest adjourned for any reason, he may, at any time before the date so fixed, alter the date, hour or place fixed and shall then give reasonable notice to the persons within paragraph (4).

(4) The persons within this paragraph are the members of the jury (if any), the witnesses, the chief officer of police, any person notified under Rule 19 or 24 and any other person appearing in person or represented at the inquest.

COMMENTARY ON RULE 33

General Note

"Where a coroner has fixed a date ..." in subrule (3). Coroner includes deputy and assistant deputy coroner: rule 2(1) *ante*, at page 38.

Forms

For the appropriate Form in the case of subrule (1) see Sched. 4, Form 15. In the case of subrule. (2) see Sched. 4, Form 16. In the case of subrule (3) see Sched. 4 Form 18, *post*, at page 71.

RULE 34

Recognizance of witness or juror becoming void

34. Where any witness or juror who has been bound over to attend at an adjourned inquest, whether without further notice or conditionally on receiving further notice, is notified by the coroner that his attendance at the adjourned inquest is not required or that the inquest will not be resumed, the recognizance entered into by him shall be void.

COMMENTARY ON RULE 34

General Note

The entering into a recognizance by witnesses is an anomaly peculiar to coroners' proceedings. It remains unreformed by the Criminal Procedure (Attendance of Witnesses) Act 1965. In practice it is rarely if ever used.

Forms

See Schedule 4, Form 17.

RULE 35

Coroner to notify Crown Court officer of adjournment in certain cases

35. Where a person charged with an offence within Rule 26(3) is committed for trial to the Crown Court, the coroner who has adjourned an inquest in pursuance of section 20 of the Act of 1926 shall inform the appropriate officer of the Crown Court at the place where the person charged is to be tried of such adjournment.

RULE 36

Matters to be ascertained at inquest

36. (1) The proceedings and evidence at an inquest shall be directed solely to ascertaining the following matters, namely

    (*a*) who the deceased was;

    (*b*) how, when and where the deceased came by his death;

    (*c*) the particulars for the time being required by the Registration Acts to be registered concerning the death.

(2) Neither the coroner nor the jury shall express any opinion on any other matters.

COMMENTARY ON RULE 36

Riders to Verdicts

It would seem that riders were never specifically authorised. They seem to have been traditional, and the 1953 Rules ordained that they must be restricted to preventing similar fatalities. The 1971 Brodrick Report, Cmnd. 4810, at page 193, para. 16.53 recommended that riders be abolished altogether. Rule 36(2) of the 1984 Rules States that "Neither the coroner nor the jury shall express any opinion on any matters [other than those set out in rule 36(1)]. However, rule 43, *post*, authorises the coroner to announce publicly that he intends to report the matter in question to the appropriate person or authority who may have power to take the necessary action to prevent similar fatalities, and to report it accordingly.

RULE 37

Documentary evidence

37. (1) Subject to the provisions of paragraphs (2) to (4), the coroner may admit at an inquest documentary evidence relevant to the purposes of the inquest from any living person which in his opinion is unlikely to be disputed, unless a person who in the opinion of the coroner is within Rule 20(2) objects to the documentary evidence being admitted.

(2) Documentary evidence so objected to may be admitted if in the opinion of the coroner the maker of the document is unable to give oral evidence within a reasonable period.

(3) Subject to paragraph (4), before admitting such documentary evidence the coroner shall at the beginning of the inquest announce publicly:

(*a*) that the documentary evidence may be admitted, and

(*b*) (i) the full name of the maker of the document to be admitted in evidence, and

(ii) a brief account of such document, and

(*c*) that any person who in the opinion of the coroner is within Rule 20(2) may object to the admission of any such documentary evidence, and

(*d*) that any person who in the opinion of the coroner is within Rule 20(2) is entitled to see a copy of any such documentary evidence if he so wishes.

(4) If during the course of an inquest it appears that there is available at the inquest documentary evidence which in the opinion of the coroner is relevant to the purposes of the inquest but the maker of the document is not present and in the opinion of the coroner the content of the documentary evidence is unlikely to be disputed, the coroner shall at the earliest opportunity during the course of the inquest comply with the provisions of paragraph (3).

(5) A coroner may admit as evidence at an inquest any document made by a deceased person if he is of the opinion that the contents of the document are relevant to the purposes of the inquest.

(6) Any documentary evidence admitted under this Rule shall, unless the coroner otherwise directs, be read aloud at the inquest.

RULE 38

Exhibits

38. All exhibits produced in evidence at an inquest shall be marked with consecutive numbers and each number shall be preceded by the letter "C."

RULE 39

Notes of evidence

39. The coroner shall take notes of the evidence at every inquest.

COMMENTARY ON RULE 39

General Note

A tape recording of proceedings satisfies the rule: *R.* v. *South London Coroner, ex parte Thompson and Others, The Times,* July 9, 1982, D.C.

RULE 40

No addresses as to facts

40. No person shall be allowed to address the coroner or the jury as to the facts.

COMMENTARY ON RULE 40

General Note

A properly interested person or his representative may address the coroner as to the law.

RULE 41

Summing-up and direction to jury

41. Where the coroner sits with a jury, he shall sum up the evidence to the jury and direct them as to the law before they consider their verdict and shall draw their attention to Rules 36(2) and 42.

RULE 42

Verdict

42. No verdict shall be framed in such a way as to appear to determine any question of

    (*a*) criminal liability on the part of a named person, or
    (*b*) civil liability.

COMMENTARY ON RULE 42

General Note

A list of suggested verdicts is set out in Schedule 4, Form 22, note 4, *post.* See the commentary thereto, *post* at page 74. The coroner may make recommendations (either on his own initiative or that of the jury) but these are not part of the verdict; see rule 43.

See *R.* v. *Walthamstow Coroner, ex parte Rubenstein* [1982] Crim L.R. 509, D.C., where it was said, *obiter,* that a verdict which included the words "aggravated by neglect" was a verdict which could be reached without breach of rule 53(*b*) of the 1953 Rules (rule 42 of the 1984 Rules is the new equivalent of the old rule 53 which prohibited verdicts determining questions of civil liability) as it did not specifically refer to a particular person. See *R.* v. *Surrey Coroner, ex parte Campbell* [1982] 2 W.L.R. 626; [1982] 2 All E.R. 545, D.C.: a verdict of lack of care by another or others did not transgress the requirement under r.33(*b*) of the Coroners Rules 1953 (now rule 42(*b*)).

Further, see note 24a, *ante,* at page 21 and commentary on Schedule 4, Form 22, 1984 Rules, *post,* at page 74.

Forms

See Schedule 4, Form 22, *post.*

RULE 43

Prevention of similar fatalities

43. A coroner who believes that action should be taken to prevent the recurrence of fatalities similar to that in respect of which the inquest is being held may announce at the inquest that he is reporting the matter in writing to the person or authority who may have power to take such action and he may report the matter accordingly.

COMMENTARY ON RULE 43

General Note

Rule 34 of the 1953 Rules, which permitted riders designed to prevent the recurrence of similar fatalities, was repealed by the Coroners (Amendment) Rules 1980 (S.I. 1980 No. 557), which substituted what is now rule 43 of the 1984 Rules.

RULE 44

Summoning of jurors

44. Subject to the provisions of these Rules, the person to whom the coroner's warrant is issued under section 3 of the Act of 1887 for the summoning of persons to attend as jurors at inquests shall have regard to the convenience of the persons summoned and to their respective places of residence, and in particular to the desirability of selecting jurors within reasonable daily travelling distance of the place where they are to attend.

COMMENTARY ON RULE 44

Women Jurors

A prior decision or custom to exclude women from the jury is wrong: *R.* v. *Surrey Coroner, ex parte Campbell,* [1982] Q.B. 661; [1982] 2 All E.R. 545.

Forms

For Jurors' Oath see Schedule 4, Form 7, *post*, at page 68.

RULE 45

Method of summoning

45. Subject to the provisions of these Rules, jurors shall be summoned by notice in writing sent by post or delivered by hand and a notice shall be sent or delivered to a juror at his address as shown in the electoral register.

COMMENTARY ON RULE 45

Forms

See Schedule 4, Form 4, *post*, at page 65.

RULE 46

Notice to accompany summons

46. A written summons sent or delivered to any person under Rule 45 shall be accompanied by a notice informing him—

  (*a*) of the effect of section 3A of the Act of 1887 and Rules 51(1) and 52; and
  (*b*) that he may make representations to the appropriate officer with a view to obtaining the withdrawal of the summons, if for any reason he is not qualified for jury service, or wishes or is entitled to be excused.

COMMENTARY ON RULE 46

Forms

See Schedule 4, Form 5, *post*.

RULE 47

Withdrawal or alteration of summons

47. If it appears to the appropriate officer, at any time before the day on which any person summoned under section 3 of the Act of 1887 is to attend, that his attendance is unnecessary, or can be dispensed with, the appropriate officer may withdraw or alter the summons by notice served in the same way as a notice of summons.

RULE 48

Summoning in exceptional circumstances

48. If it appears to the coroner that a jury will be, or probably will be, incomplete, the coroner may, if he thinks fit, require any persons who are in, or in the vicinity of, the place of the inquest to be summoned (without any written notice) for jury service up to the number needed (after allowing for any who may not be qualified under section 3A of the Act of 1887 and for excusals) to make up such number.

COMMENTARY ON RULE 48

General Note

See commentary to rule 44, *ante.*

RULE 49

Excusal for previous jury service

49.—(1) If a person summoned under section 3 of the Act of 1887 shows to the satisfaction of the appropriate officer or of the coroner—

    (*a*) that he has served on a jury, or duly attended to serve on a jury, at inquests held in that coroner's jurisdiction on three or more days in the period of one year ending with the service of the summons on him; or

    (*b*) that he has served on a jury, or duly attended to serve on a jury, in the Crown Court, the High Court or any county court in the period of two years ending with the service of the summons on him; or

    (*c*) that any such court or a coroner has excused him from jury service for a period which has not terminated,

the appropriate officer or the coroner shall excuse him from attending, or further attending, in pursuance of the summons.

(2) In reckoning the days for the purpose of paragraph (1)(*a*) no account shall be taken of any day or days to which an inquest is adjourned.

RULE 50

Certificate of attendance

50. A person duly attending to serve on a jury in compliance with a summons under section 3 of the Act of 1887 shall be entitled on application to the appropriate officer to a certificate recording that he has so attended.

COMMENTARY ON RULE 50

Forms

See Schedule 4, Form 6, *post.*

RULE 51

Excusal for certain persons and discretionary excusal

51.—(1) A person summoned under section 3 of the Act of 1887 shall be entitled, if he so wishes, to be excused from jury service if he is among the persons for the time being listed in Part III of Schedule 1 to the Juries Act 1974 but, except as provided by that Part of that Schedule in the case of members of the forces, a person shall not by this Rule be exempt from his obligation to attend if summoned unless he is excused from attending under paragraph (2).

(2) If any person so summoned shows to the satisfaction of the appropriate officer or of the coroner that there is good reason why he should be excused from attending in pursuance of the summons, the appropriate officer or the coroner may excuse him from so attending and shall do so if the reason shown is that the person is entitled under paragraph (1) to excusal.

RULE 52

Discharge of summons in case of doubt as to capacity to act effectively as a juror

52. Where it appears to the appropriate officer, in the case of a person attending in pursuance of a summons under section 3 of the Act of 1887, that on account of physical disability or insufficient understanding of English there is doubt as to his capacity to act effectively as a juror, the person may be brought before the coroner, who shall determine whether or not he should act as a juror and, if not, shall discharge the summons.

RULE 53

Saving for inquests held by the coroner of the Queen's household

53. Nothing in this Part of these Rules shall have effect in relation to any inquest held by the coroner of the Queen's household.

RULE 54

Register of deaths

54. A coroner shall keep an indexed register of all deaths reported to him, or to his deputy or assistant deputy, which shall contain the particulars specified in Schedule 3.

RULE 55

Retention and delivery or disposal of exhibits

55. Every exhibit at an inquest shall, unless a court otherwise directs, be retained by the coroner until he is satisfied that the exhibit is not likely to be, or will no longer be, required for the purposes of any other legal proceedings, and shall then, if a request for its delivery has been made by a person appearing to the coroner to be entitled to the possession thereof, be delivered to that person, or, if no such request has been made, be destroyed or otherwise disposed of as the coroner thinks fit.

RULE 56

Retention and delivery of documents

56. Any document (other than an exhibit at an inquest) in the possession of a coroner in connection with an inquest or post-mortem examination shall, unless a court otherwise directs, be retained by the coroner for at least fifteen years:

Provided that the coroner may deliver any such document to any person who in the opinion of the coroner is a proper person to have possession of it.

RULE 57

Inspection of, or supply of copies of, documents etc.

57. (1) A coroner shall, on application and on payment of the prescribed fee (if any), supply to any person who, in the opinion of the coroner, is a properly interested person a copy of any report of a post-mortem examination (including one made under section 21 of the Act of 1926) or special examination, or of any notes of evidence, or of any document put in evidence at an inquest.

(2) A coroner may, on application and without charge, permit any person who, in the opinion of the coroner, is a properly interested person to inspect such report, notes of evidence, or document.

COMMENTARY ON RULE 57

General Note

"Permit any person . . . to inspect." The right to inspect also carries with it the right to copy: *Nelson* v. *Anglo-American Land Mortgage Co.* [1897] 1 Ch. 130.

RULE 58

Deputy or assistant deputy to sign documents in own name

58. Where a deputy or assistant deputy coroner acting for, or as, the coroner signs a document, he shall sign it in his own name as deputy or assistant deputy coroner, as the case may be.

RULE 59

Transfer of documents etc. to next-appointed coroner

59. Where a coroner vacates his office by death or otherwise, all documents, exhibits, registers and other things in the custody of the coroner in connection with inquests or post-mortem examinations shall be transferred to the coroner next appointed to that office.

RULE 60

Forms

60. The forms set out in Schedule 4, with such modifications as circumstances may require, may be used for the purposes for which they are expressed to be applicable.

SCHEDULES

SCHEDULE 1

REVOCATIONS

Rules Revoked	References
The Coroners Rules 1953	S.I. 1953/205
The Coroners Rules 1956	S.I. 1956/1691
The Coroners (Amendment) Rules 1974	S.I. 1974/2128
The Coroners (Amendment) Rules 1977	S.I. 1977/1881
The Coroners (Amendment) Rules 1980	S.I. 1980/557
The Coroners (Amendment) (Savings) Rules 1980	S.I. 1980/668
The Coroners (Amendment) Rules 1983	S.I. 1983/1539

SCHEDULE 2 **Rule 10**

POST–MORTEM EXAMINATION REPORT

THIS REPORT IS CONFIDENTIAL. IT SHOULD NOT BE DISCLOSED TO A THIRD PARTY WITHOUT THE CORONER'S CONSENT

POST-MORTEM EXAMINATION REPORT Serial No.:
Name of deceased: Coroner:
Address (if known):
Identified by: Place of examination: Date and time of examination:
Observers present at examination:

EXTERNAL EXAMINATION[1]

Stated/Estimated date and time of death: Stated/Apparent age:
Nourishment:
Marks of identification (tattoos, old scars, etc.):
Body surface and musculo-skeletal system, including injuries:

INTERNAL EXAMINATION[1]

Central nervous system

Cranial
cavity
{ Skull:
Brain:
Meninges:
Cerebral vessels:

Respiratory system[2]

Thoracic
cavity
{ Larynx:
Trachea:
Bronchi:
Pleurae:
Lung parenchyma:

Cardio-vascular system
Heart:
  Weight:
  Valves:
  Myocardium:
  Pericardium:
  Coronary arteries:
  Great vessels:

Alimentary system
Mouth:
Tongue:
Oesophagus:

Abdominal
cavity
{ Stomach and contents:
Duodenum:
Intestines:
Liver and gall bladder:
Pancreas:
Peritoneum:

Genito-urinary system
Kidneys and ureters:
Bladder and urine:
Generative organs:

Reticulo-endothelial system
Spleen:
Lymph nodes:
Thymus:

Endocrine system
Thyroid:
Pituitary:
Adrenals:

In my opinion the cause of death was:

I	I

Disease or condition   (a) ....
directly leading to   due to (or as a consequence of)
death[3]

Antecedent causes.   (b) ....
  Morbid conditions,   due to (or as a consequence of)
  if any, giving rise
  to the above cause
  (stating the underlying
  condition last)   (c) ....

II	II

Other significant conditions
contributing to the death
but NOT related to the
disease or condition
causing it[4]
                           ....

Morbid conditions present but in the
pathologist's opinion *NOT contributing to the death:*

Is any further laboratory examination to be made which may affect the
cause of death? YES/NO

Comments:

To the best of my knowledge no cardiac pacemaker remains in the body.
Signature and qualifications
Name (in block letters)

Notes

[1] Descriptions of injuries or of complex pathology may be attached on a separate
sheet, provided it is properly identified and signed.

[2] In cases of suspected pneumoconiosis (or one of the other occupational diseases
affecting the lungs) see "Notes on completing the post-mortem examination report
form" obtainable from the coroner.

[3] This does not mean the mode of dying, such as (*e.g.*) heart failure, asphyxia, asthenia, etc. It means the disease, injury or complication which caused death.

[4] Conditions which did not in the pathologist's opinion contribute materially to the death should *not* be included under this heading, but under "Morbid conditions present but in the pathologist's opinion *not* contributing to the death."

SCHEDULE 3   Rule 54

REGISTER OF DEATHS REPORTED TO THE CORONER

Date on which death is reported to coroner	Particulars of deceased		Cause of death	State whether case disposed of by using Pink Form A or B or whether inquest was held	Verdict at inquest (if any)
	Full name and address	Age Sex			

SCHEDULE 4   Rule 60

FORMS

1

Form of declaration of office of coroner

I, A.B., solemnly, sincerely, and truly declare and affirm that I will well and truly serve our Sovereign Lady the Queen and Her liege people in the office of coroner for this county of   , and that I will diligently and truly do everything appertaining to my office to the best of my power for the doing of right, and for the good of the inhabitants within the said county.

2

Warrant to exhume

To

(*insert the names of the Minister and churchwardens or other persons having power of control over the churchyard, cemetery, or other place in which the body is buried*).

Whereas I, A.B., one of Her Majesty's coroners for the   of
       am credibly informed that the body of one, C.D., has been
recently buried in   *(insert the name of the churchyard, cemetery or
other place in which the body is buried)* , and it appears to me that it is necessary for the
body to be examined for the purpose of [my holding an inquest touching the death of
the deceased] [my discharging one of my functions in relation to the body or death of
the deceased, namely *(insert function)*:

I hereby order you to cause the body of the said C.D. to be disinterred for that
purpose.

    Dated this   day of   19 .

                         Signature ....
                         Coroner for ....

3

Warrant to summon jury

To the Coroner's officer and to each and all of the constables of   .
You are hereby commanded to summon   jurors to appear before me on
           (state day of week) the   *(state date)* day of
          19 , at   a.m./p.m. at   *(state place).*

    Dated this   day of   19 .

                         Signature ....
                         Coroner for ....

4

Summons to juror

To
By virtue of a warrant of A.B., one of Her Majesty's coroners for the
         of   you are hereby summoned to appear before
him as a juror on   *(state day of week)* the   *(state
date)* day of   19 , at   a.m./p.m. at   *(state place)*
until you are no longer needed.

    You must attend at the time and place shown above unless you are told by the
officer authorised by the Coroner that you need not do so.

    Dated this   day of   19 .

                         Signature ....
                         Coroner's Officer/Constable ....

YOU MUST COMPLETE THE ATTACHED FORM AND RETURN IT TO
(insert name of officer authorised by the Coroner) IN THE ENVELOPE PROVIDED
WITHIN THREE DAYS OF THE RECEIPT OF THIS SUMMONS.

WARNING: YOU WILL BE LIABLE TO A FINE IF YOU—

    1. refuse to give the information necessary to decide if you are qualified to serve
       on a jury;

2. deliberately give false information or cause or permit false information to be given;
3. fail to attend for jury service or refuse without reasonable excuse to serve as a juror; or
4. serve on a jury knowing you are not qualified to do so.

5

Notice to accompany summons and reply thereto

This form should be returned in the envelope provided within three days of receiving it.

Surname ....

Forename(s) .... Date of Birth ....

Address ....

.... Telephone number ....
(If possible please give a telephone number where you can be contacted between 9 a.m. and 5 p.m.)

INFORMATION GIVEN WILL BE TREATED IN THE STRICTEST CONFIDENCE

YOU ARE QUALIFIED for jury service if you—

(a) are over eighteen and under sixty-five;

[If you will be under eighteen on or have reached your sixty-fifth birthday by the date on which your appearance is required you will NOT be eligible to serve as a juror.]

(b) are registered as a parliamentary or local government elector;
(c) have lived in the United Kingdom, the Channel Islands or the Isle of Man for a period of at least five years since attaining the age of thirteen; and

(d) are not one of the persons described in Parts I and II of Schedule 1 to the Juries Act 1974.*

1. Are you QUALIFIED to serve as a juror? Please tick appropriate box.

YES ☐   NO ☐

If you have answered NO to question 1, please answer question 2 and sign the form at the end.

If you have answered YES and wish to apply to be excused from jury service on this occasion, please go on to 3 below and then sign the form at the end.

2. I AM NOT QUALIFIED to serve on a jury because—

3. YOU ARE ENTITLED TO BE EXCUSED if you fall within any of the categories of persons specified in Part III of Schedule 1 to the Juries Act 1974† (although you may serve if you want to).

YOU MAY BE EXCUSED at the discretion of the Coroner or of the officer authorised by the Coroner on grounds such as poor health, illness, physical disability, insufficient understanding of English, holiday arrangements or for any other good reason.

I WISH TO BE EXCUSED from jury service on this occasion because—

[If you are in any doubt as to whether you may be excused from jury service please write to the officer authorised by the Coroner at the address on the front of the summons.]

When you attend as a juror you may be discharged if there is doubt as to your capacity to serve on a jury because of physical disability or insufficient understanding of English.

I HAVE READ THE WARNING IN THE SUMMONS AND THE INFORMATION I HAVE GIVEN IS TRUE.

Signed .... Dated ....

*See List 1 attached.
†See List 2 attached.

6

Certificate of attendance

Name of Juror ....

I hereby certify that the above-named Juror [attended to serve] [served] on a jury at an inquest held before A.B., one of Her Majesty's coroners for the
of

*Delete as   *on/*from
 required   *to

[and I further certify that in the opinion of the Coroner it would be reasonable and proper that he/she should be exempt from service on a jury in a coroner's court for a period of   years from   .]

Dated this   day of   19 .

Signature ....
Officer authorised by the Coroner.

67

7

Form of oath of juror

I swear by Almighty God that I will diligently inquire and a true presentment make of all such matters and things as are here given me in charge on behalf of our Sovereign Lady the Queen, touching the death of C.D., now lying dead, and will, without fear or favour, affection or ill-will, a true verdict give according to the evidence.

NOTE: If a person wishes to affirm, or swear in Scottish form or in any other form authorised by law, this oath shall be modified accordingly.

8

Summons to witness

To

You are hereby summoned to appear before me on   *(state day of week)* the   *(state date)* day of   19 , at   a.m./p.m., at   *(state place)* to give evidence touching the death of C.D.

Dated this   day of   19 .

Signature ....
Coroner for ....

9

Oath of witness

I swear by Almighty God that the evidence which I shall give shall be the truth, the whole truth and nothing but the truth.

NOTE: If a person wishes to affirm, or swear in Scottish form or in any other form authorised by law, this oath shall be modified accordingly.

10

Direction to medical practitioner to make a post-mortem examination

To

I hereby direct you, in pursuance of section 21 of the [Coroners Act 1887] [Coroners (Amendment) Act 1926], to make a post-mortem examination of the body of C.D. and to report the result thereof to me in writing.

Dated this   day of   19 .

Signature ....
Coroner for ....

11

Certificate of fine

I hereby certify that I have imposed a fine of   upon E.F. for that
he being duly summoned to appear as a juror [witness] at an inquest held before [by]
me on the   day of   19 ,
*Delete as   *did not, after being openly called three times, appear to such summons.
required   *refused, without reasonable excuse, to serve as a juror.
             *refused, without lawful excuse, to answer a question put to him.

Dated this   day of   19 .

Signature ....
Coroner for ....

12

Form of recognizance—witnesses or jurors

G.H. of   acknowledges that he/she owes to our Sovereign Lady
the Queen the sum of   , payment thereof to be enforced against
him/her by due process of law if he/she fails to comply with the following condition.

Taken before me the   day of   19 .

Signature ....
Coroner for ....

Condition

If the said G.H. [on receiving notice] appears at an inquest touching the death of
C.D. to be held on the   day of   next at
                    , or on such other date or at such other place as may be notified to
him/her, and there gives evidence [makes further inquiry as a juror] touching the
said death, then this recognizance shall be void but otherwise shall remain in full
force.

13

Notice of inquest arrangements

To
I hereby give you notice that the inquest touching the death of C.D. will take place
on   *(state day of week)* the   *(state date)* day of
                    19 , at   a.m./p.m. at   *(state*
place).

Dated this   day of   19 .

Signature ....
Coroner for ....

14

Coroner's interim certificate of the fact of death

To whom it may concern.

(Name) ....

of (address) ....

....

died on ....

The precise medical cause of death *was as follows/*has yet to be established.

....

Dated this   day of   19 .

                     Signature ....

                     Coroner for ....

*Delete whichever is inapplicable.

15

Notice that an inquest which is adjourned in pursuance of section 20 of the Coroners (Amendment) Act 1926 will not be resumed

To

I hereby give you notice that the inquest touching the death of C.D. will not be resumed.

Dated this   day of   19 .

                     Signature ....

                     Coroner for ....

16

Notice that an inquest which is adjourned in pursuance of section 20 of the Coroners (Amendment) Act 1926 will be resumed

To

I hereby give you notice that the inquest touching the death of C.D. will be resumed on   *(state day of week)* the   *(state date)* day of   19   at   a.m./p.m. at
            (state place) [and that your attendance thereat is required].

Dated this   day of   19 .

                     Signature ....

                     Coroner for ....

17

Notice that the attendance of a witness will not be required at the holding of an adjourned inquest

To

I hereby give you notice that your attendance at the adjourned inquest touching the death of C.D. to be held on the   day of
19   , will not be required.

‘ Dated this   day of   19   .

Signature ....
Coroner for ....

18

Notice that the date, hour or place fixed for the holding of an adjourned inquest has been altered

To

I hereby give you notice that the date/hour/place fixed for the holding of the adjourned inquest touching the death of C.D. has been altered, and that the adjourned inquest will be held on   *(state date and day of week)* at
a.m./p.m. at   *(state place)* [and that your attendance thereat is/is not required].

Dated this   day of   19   .

Signature ....
Coroner for ....

19

Certificate of forfeiture of recognizance

I hereby certify that G.H. of   was bound by recognizance taken by
me on the   day of   19   , in the sum of
for his appearance at an inquest held at   on the
day of   19   , to give evidence [make further inquiry as a juror] touching the death of C.D., and the said G.H. failed to appear in accordance with the condition of the said recognizance and that the said recognizance is accordingly forfeited.

Dated this   day of   19   .

Signature ....
Coroner for ....

20

Order to remove body for inquest or post-mortem examination

To   *(undertaker or other person as the case may be)* I hereby
authorise you to remove the body of C.D., aged   from
                     to   before the   day of
                     19   .

Dated this   day of   19   .

Signature ....
Coroner for ....

21

Coroner's order for burial

I hereby authorise the burial of the body of C.D. aged   late of
                     who died at   on   .

Dated this   day of   19   .

Signature ....
Coroner for ....

22

Inquisition

An inquisition taken for our Sovereign Lady the Queen at   , in
the county *(or as the case may be)* of   on the
day of   19   , [and by adjournment on the   day
of   19   ,] [before and by [1]] me A.B., one of Her Majesty's coroners
for the said county *(or as the case may be)*, [and the undermentioned jurors,] touching
the death of C.D. [a person unknown]   [concerning a stillbirth].

The following matters are found:—

1. Name of deceased (if known):
2. Injury or disease causing death:[2]
3. Time, place and circumstances at or in which injury was sustained:[3]
4. Conclusion of the jury/coroner as to the death:[4]
5. Particulars for the time being required by the Registration Acts to be registered
   concerning the death:

(1) Date and place of death	(2) Name and surname of deceased	(3) Sex	(4) Maiden surname of woman who has married	(5) Date and place of birth	(6) Occupation and usual address

Signature of coroner [and jurors] ....

Notes

[1] Modify this as necessary according to whether the inquest is held with or without a jury or partly with and partly without a jury.

[2] In the case of a death from natural causes or from industrial disease, want of attention at birth, or dependence on, or non-dependent abuse of, drugs insert the immediate cause of death and the morbid conditions (if any) giving rise to the immediate cause of death.

[3] Omit this if the cause of death is one to which Note 2 applies.

[4] (*a*) Where the cause of death is one to which Note 2 applies, it is suggested that one of the following forms be adopted:—

> C.D. died from natural causes.
> C.D. died from the industrial disease of
> C.D. died from dependence on drugs/non-dependent abuse of drugs.
> C.D. died from want of attention at birth.

> (In any of the above cases, but in no other, it is suggested that the following words may, where appropriate, be added:
> "and the cause of death was aggravated by lack of care/self neglect".)

(*b*) In any other case except murder, manslaughter, infanticide or stillbirth, it is suggested that one of the following forms be adopted:—

> C.D. killed himself [whilst the balance of his mind was disturbed].
> C.D. died as a result of an attempted/self-induced abortion.
> C.D. died as a result of an accident/misadventure.
> Execution of sentence of death.
> C.D. was killed lawfully.
> Open verdict, namely, the evidence did not fully or further disclose the means whereby the cause of death arose.

(*c*) In the case of murder, manslaughter or infanticide it is suggested that the following form be adopted:—

> C.D. was killed unlawfully.

(*d*) In the case of a stillbirth insert "stillbirth" and do not complete the remainder of the form.

73

COMMENTARY ON FORM 22

General Note

Open Verdict. An open verdict is, generally speaking, undesirable. However, if there is insufficient evidence to record any of the other suggested verdicts, an open verdict may be recorded. The fact that there may be uncertainty regarding some minor point or *e.g.* the precise cause, place or time of death, does not authorise recording an open verdict if there is sufficient evidence to record how the deceased came by his death. See also the remarks of the Divisional Court in *R.* v. *City of London Coroner, ex parte Barber* [1975] 1 W.L.R. 1310 at p. 1313 and *R.* v. *Southwark Coroner, ex parte Calvi, The Times,* April 2, 1983.

Suicide. To support a verdict of suicide there should be some actual evidence pointing to the event and the verdict should not rest upon surmise: *R.* v. *Huntbach, ex parte Lockley* [1944] K.B. 606. Suicide must be strictly proved at an inquest; it is not a verdict which should be reached as being the most likely cause of death: *R.* v. *City of London Coroner, ex parte Barber* [1975] 1 W.L.R. 1310; [1975] 3 All E.R. 538, D.C. Satisfactory evidence of suicidal intent is always necessary to establish suicide as the cause of death: *R.* v. *Cardiff Coroner, ex parte Thomas* [1970] 3 All E.R. 469, D.C. (*Re Davis* [1967] 2 W.L.R. 1089 distinguished).

"C.D. was killed unlawfully." By the Criminal Law Act 1977, s.56(1) a coroner's inquisition shall in no case charge a person with an offence of murder, manslaughter or infanticide.

"Lack of care/self neglect." See commentary on rule 42, *ante,* at p. 55. In the unreported inquest of *Michael Martin, dec'd.* (held at Bracknell Crown Court on October 4, 1984), the coroner directed the jury that, notwithstanding the suggestion regarding "lack of care" verdicts in Schedule 4 of the 1984 Rules, it was open to them to return the verdict "accidental death aggravated by lack of care" where the death had occurred in custody at Broadmoor. The coroner did so after hearing submissions by counsel to the effect that:

(1) The suggestion in the Schedule to the Rules was merely a suggestion.

(2) The Rules being in the form of a Statutory Instrument could not override an actual Statute.

(3) The Coroners Act 1887 laid upon the jury the duty of inquiring into how, in the fullest sense, someone had died. The judgment of the Divisional Court in *R.* v. *H.M. Coroner for Surrey, ex p. Campbell, ante* had made that clear.

This decision, that of a coroner, is not binding.

THE CORONERS ACTS

The Coroners Act 1844 (c. 92)
The Coroners Act 1887 (c. 71)
The Coroners Act 1892 (c. 56)
The Coroners (Amendment) Act 1926 (c. 59)
The Coroners Act 1954 (c. 31)
The Coroners Act 1980 (c. 38)

THE CORONERS ACT 1844

(7 & 8 Vict. c. 92)

An Act to amend the law respecting the Officer of County Coroner.

[9th August 1844]

SECTION 2 [Repealed]

[2.]

SECTION 3 [Repealed]

[3.]

SECTION 4 [Repealed]

[4.]

Note. Sections 2, 3 and 4 were repealed by the Coroners (Amendment) Act, 1926, s.31 and Schedule 3. However, s.31 of *ibid.* provides:

> "Any Order in Council made under section four of the Coroners Act, 1844, shall continue in force and shall have effect as if it were an order providing for the division of a county into coroners' districts or for the alteration of an existing division of a county into coroners' districts or for the alteration of an existing division of a county into coroners' districts, as the case may be, made by the Secretary of State under this Act."

SECTION 5

Districts to be assigned to coroners

5. The justices in general or quarter session assembled shall assign one of such districts to each of the persons holding the office of coroner in such county, and upon the death, resignation, or removal of any such person, each of his successors, and also every other person thereafter elected into the office of coroner in such county, [. . .] shall exercise the office of coroner, according to the provisions of this act [. . .].

COMMENTARY ON SECTION 5

Amendments

The words omitted in the first set of square brackets were repealed by the Statute Law Reform Act, 1891.

The words omitted in the second set of square brackets were repealed by the Local Government Act 1972, s.220(5) and Schedule 30.

General Note

See the Coroners (Amendment) Act, 1926, s.12(4), *post.*

SECTION 19

Coroner elected for a district to be coroner for the whole County

19. Every coroner elected under the authority of this act, although such coroner may be designated as the coroner for any particular district of a county, [...] shall for all purposes whatsoever, except as hereinafter mentioned, be considered as a coroner for the whole county, and shall have the same jurisdiction, rights, powers, and authorities throughout the said county as if he had been elected one of the coroners of said county [...].

COMMENTARY ON SECTION 19

Amendments

The words omitted were repealed by the Statute Law Reform Act, 1891.

General Note

See the 1926 Act, s.12(4), *post,* at page 107.

SECTION 20

Coroners (except during illness, etc.) to hold inquests only within the district to which they are assigned—coroner holding inquest elsewhere to certify the reason

20. [...] [Except as aforesaid, every coroner for any county, or any district thereof, or his deputy, after he shall, in pursuance of the provisions of this Act, have been assigned to [...] any particular district, shall, except during illness or incapacity or unavoidable absence as aforesaid of any coroner for any other district, or during a vacancy in the office of coroner for any other district, hold inquests only within the district to or for which he shall have been assigned [...] Provided always, that the coroner who shall, by himself or deputy, hold any inquest in any other district save that to which he shall have been assigned [. . .] as aforesaid shall, in his inquisition to be returned on such inquest, certify the cause of his attendance and holding such inquest; which certificate shall be conclusive evidence of the illness or incapacity or unavoidable absence as aforesaid of the coroner in whose stead he shall so attend, or of there being a vacancy in the office of coroner for the district in which such inquest shall be holden.

COMMENTARY ON SECTION 20

Amendments

The words omitted were repealed by the Statute Law Reform Act 1891.

General Note

The Coroners Act 1980, s.2(1), *post*, confers on a coroner the power to transfer jurisidiction to a coroner in another area without requiring the body to be moved into the area of the coroner who is to hold the inquest.

See the 1926 Act, s.12(4), *post*, at page 107.

SECTION 27 [Repealed]

[27.]

Note. Section 27 was repealed by the local Government Act, 1972, Schedule 30.

THE CORONERS ACT 1887

(50 & 51 Vict. c. 71)

An Act to consolidate the law relating to Coroners.

[16th September 1887]

PART I

SECTION 1

Short Title

1. This Act may be cited as the Coroners Act 1887.

SECTION 2

Extent of Act

2. This Act shall not apply to Scotland or Ireland.

SECTION 3

Summoning and swearing of jury by Coroner

3. (1) Where a coroner is informed that the dead body of a person is lying within his jurisdiction, and there is reasonable cause to suspect that such person has died either a violent or an unnatural death, or has died a sudden death of which the cause is unknown, or that such person has died in prison, or in such place or under such circumstances as to require an inquest in pursuance of any Act, the coroner, whether the cause of death arose within his jurisdiction or not, shall, as soon as practicable, issue his warrant for summoning not less than [seven nor more than eleven] good and lawful men to appear before him at a specified time and place, there to inquire as jurors touching the death of such person as aforesaid.

(2) Where an inquest is held [touching the death] of a prisoner who dies within a prison, [...] a prisoner therein or a person engaged in any sort of trade or dealing with the prison shall not be a juror on such inquest.

(3) When not less than [seven] jurors are assembled they shall be sworn by or before the coroner diligently to inquire touching the death [...] and a true verdict to give according to the evidence.

"Qualifications of jurors

[**3A.** (1) A person shall not be qualified to serve as a juror at an inquest held by a coroner unless he is for the time being qualified to serve as a juror in the Crown Court, the High Court and county courts in accordance with section 1 of the Juries Act 1974.

(2) If a person serves on a jury knowing that he is ineligible for such service under Group A, B or C in Part I of Schedule 1 to that Act he shall be guilty of an offence and liable on summary conviction to a fine not exceeding level 3 on the standard scale.

(3) If a person serves on a jury knowing that he is disqualified for such service under Part II of that Schedule he shall be guilty of an offence and liable on summary conviction to a fine not exceeding level 5 on the standard scale.

(4) The appropriate officer may at any time put or cause to be put to any person who is summoned under section 3 of this Act such questions as he thinks fit in order to establish whether or not the person is qualified to serve as a juror at an inquest.

(5) Where a question is put to any person under subsection (4) of this section, if that person refuses without reasonable excuse to answer, or gives an answer which he knows to be false in a material particular, or recklessly gives an answer which is false in a material particular, he shall be guilty of an offence and liable on summary conviction to a fine not exceeding level 3 on the standard scale.

(6) If any person

(a) duly summoned as a juror at an inquest makes, or causes or permits to be made on his behalf, any false representation to the coroner or the appropriate officer with the intention of evading service as such juror; or

(b) makes or causes to be made on behalf of another person who has been so summoned any false representation to the coroner or the appropriate officer with the intention of enabling that other person to evade such service;

he shall be guilty of an offence and liable on summary conviction to a fine not exceeding level 3 on the standard scale.

(7) A coroner may authorise a person to perform the functions conferred on the appropriate officer by subsection (4) of this section and references in this section to the appropriate officer shall be construed as references to the person so authorised.

(8) In this section "the standard scale" has the meaning given by section 75 of the Criminal Justice Act 1982."]

COMMENTARY ON SECTION 3

Amendments

In subsection (1) the words in square brackets were substituted by the Coroners (Amendment) Act 1926, s.30 and Schedule 2.

In subsection (2) the words in square brackets were substituted by the Coroners Act 1980, Schedule 1, para. 1.

The words omitted in subsection (2) were repealed by the Coroners Juries Act 1983, s.3(3).

In subsection (3) the word in square brackets was substituted by the Coroners (Amendment) Act 1926, s.30 and Schedule 2.

In subsection (3) the words omitted were repealed by the Coroners Act 1980, Schedule 2.

Section 3A was added by the Coroners' Juries Act, 1983, s.1.

General Note

"Within his jurisdiction" in section 3(1): the Coroner has no jurisdiction on the high seas. The sea boundary of a county extends only to the low-water mark. See *R* v. *Keyn* (1876) 2 Ex. D. 63 at p. 162. Note that it is only necessary for the body to be lying within his jurisdiction; the death may have occurred outside his jurisdiction, even outside England and Wales: *R.* v. *West Yorkshire Coroner, ex parte Smith* [1982] 3 W.L.R. 920; [1982] 3 All E.R. 1098.

Summoning a jury. For the cases in which a coroner may sit without a jury see the Coroners (Amendment) Act 1926, s.13, *post*. For the rules governing summoning of juries see The Coroners Rules 1984 (S.I. 1984 No. 552), rules 44 – 47, *ante*, at pages 55 – 57.

"Reasonable cause to suspect" in section 3(1); see: *R.* v. *Kent Justices* (1809), 11 East 229; *R.* v. *Carmarthenshire Justices* [1847], 10 Q.B. 796; *R.* v. *Stephenson* [1884], 13 Q.B.D. 331.

"As soon as practicable" in section 3(1). In practice it is now usual to open the inquest as soon as is practicable after the death, taking formal evidence of identification and such medical evidence as may be available, but the inquest is very often not completed until some time later because of the need for scientific tests and analyses, police enquiries, etc.

"Jurors." Excluding women from jury service is improper: *R.* v. *Surrey Coroner, ex parte Campbell* [1982] Q.B. 661; [1982] 2 All E.R. 545.

Section 3(1) sets out the circumstances in which a coroner is obliged to hold an inquest. Section 7(1) merely specifies which coroner is obliged to hold an inquest: *R.* v. *West Yorkshire Coroner, ex parte Smith* [1982] 3 All E.R. 1098, C.A.

SECTION 4

Proceedings at inquest—evidence and inquisition

4. (1) The coroner [. . .] shall, at the first sitting of the inquest [. . .] examine on oath touching the death all persons who tender their evidence respecting the facts and all persons having knowledge of the facts whom he thinks it expedient to examine.

[(2).]

(3) After [. . .] hearing the evidence the jury shall give their verdict, and certify it by an inquisition in writing, setting forth, so far as such particulars have been proved to them, who the deceased was, and how, when, and where the deceased came by his death [. . .]

(4) They shall also inquire of and find the particulars for the time being required by the Registration Acts to be registered concerning the death.

[(5).]

COMMENTARY ON SECTION 4

Amendments

In subsection (1) the words omitted in square brackets were repealed by the 1926 Act, s.31 and Schedule 3.

Subsection (2) was repealed by The Criminal Law Act 1977, s.65(5) and Schedules 12 and 13.

In subsection (3) the words omitted in the first square brackets were repealed by the 1926 Act, s.31 and Schedule 3. The words omitted in the second square brackets were repealed by the Criminal Law Act 1967, s.10(2) and Part III of Schedule 3 and by the Criminal Law Act 1977, s.65(5) and Schedule 13.

Subsection (5) was repealed by the 1926 Act.

General Note

"Tender their evidence" in section 4(1). The Coroner may hear evidence which would not strictly be admissible at a criminal trial (see *per* Wills J., *The Times*, March 18, 1890.

"Verdict" in section 4(3): see S.I. 1984 No. 552, Schedule 4, Form of Inquisition, Note 4, *ante* and commentary thereto at pages 72–74.

"Inquisition in writing" in section 4(3). The relevant form is found in S.I. 1984 No. 552, Schedule 4, Form 22, *ante*, at page 71.

The coroner is only permitted to communicate with the jury in open court during an inquest: *R.* v. *Reynolds* [1945] K.B. 20. Further, see note 24a, *ante*, at page 21.

SECTION 5 [Repealed]

[5.]

Note. Section 5 was repealed by the Criminal Law Act 1977, s.65(5) and Schedule 13.

SECTION 6

Ordering of coroner to hold inquest

6. (1) Where Her Majesty's High Court of Justice, upon application made by or under the authority of the Attorney General, is satisfied either—

(*a*) that a coroner refuses or neglects to hold an inquest which ought to be held; or

(*b*) where an inquest has been held by a coroner that by reason of fraud, rejection of evidence, irregularity of proceedings, insufficiency of inquiry, or otherwise, it is necessary or desirable, in the interests of justice, that another inquest should be held,

the court may order an inquest to be held touching the said death, and may, if the court think it just, order the said coroner to pay such costs of and incidental to the application as to the court may seem just, and where an inquest has been already held may quash the inquisition on that inquest.

(2) The court may order that such inquest shall be held either by the said coroner, or by any other coroner for the county, [. . .] and the coroner ordered to hold the inquest shall for that purpose have the same powers and jurisdiction as, and be deemed to be, the said coroner.

[(3).]

(4) Any power vested by this section in Her Majesty's High Court [. . .] may, subject to any rules of court made in pursuance of the Supreme Court of Judicature Act, 1875, and the Acts amending the same, be exercised by any judge of that court.

COMMENTARY ON SECTION 6

Amendments

The words omitted in subsection (2) were repealed by the Local Government Act 1972, s.272(1) and Schedule 30.

Subsection (3) was repealed by the Coroners Act 1980, s.1 and Schedule 2.

The words omitted in subsection (4) were repealed by the Statute Law Revision Act 1908.

General Note

Discovery of new facts or evidence may be grounds for quashing an inquisition and ordering a fresh inquest: the Coroners (Amendment) Act 1926, s.19 and commentary thereto, *post*, at page 111.

"Under the authority of the Attorney General" in section 6(1). The authority of the Solicitor-General will suffice in circumstances set out in the Law Officers Act 1944, s.1.

"May quash the inquisition" in section 6(1). For examples see Halsbury's *Laws of England*, Vol. 9 (4th ed.), paras. 1144 *et seq.*

The Attorney General's fiat does not dispense with the need to seek the leave of the court: *R. v. South London Coroner, ex parte Thompson and Another, The Times*, July 9, 1982, *ante*, at page 23.

Note that the same coroner "or any other coroner for the county" may hold the fresh inquest.

The Coroner's Court is also fully subject to judicial review (without the authorisation of the Attorney General but with the leave of the court) by the Divisional Court. "Since *Anisminic*, the requirements that an error of law within the jurisdiction had to appear on the face of the record was now obsolete," *per* Goff L.J. in *R. v. Greater Manchester Coroner, ex parte Tal and Another, The Times*, May 28, 1984, overruling *R. v. Surrey Coroner, ex parte Campbell* [1982] Q.B. 661.

For the alternative judicial review procedure and grounds, see *ante*, at page 23 and note 34 thereto.

SECTION 7

Local jurisdiction of coroner

7. (1) [Unless he has assumed jurisdiction under section 2 of the Coroners Act 1980] the coroner only within whose jurisdiction the body of a person upon whose death an inquest ought to be holden is lying shall hold the inquest. [...]

[(2).]

[(3).]

COMMENTARY ON SECTION 7

Amendments

In subsection (1) the words in square brackets were substituted by the Coroners Act 1980, s.3(4).

The words omitted in subsection (1) were repealed by the Coroners (Amendment) Act 1926, s.30 and Schedule 2.

Subsections (2) and (3) were repealed by the Local Government Act 1972, s.272(1) and Schedule 30.

General Note

"Jurisdiction" in section 7. Where the matters specified in section 3(3) have taken place, the coroner is under no duty to ensure that the death or cause of death occurred in England or Wales. The Coroner therefore has jurisdiction to hold an inquest: *R. v. West Yorkshire Coroner, ex parte Smith* [1982] 3 All E.R. 1098.

Section 2 of the Coroners Act 1980, *post*, at page 122, empowers a coroner to transfer his jurisdiction to hold an inquest to a coroner in another area without moving the body to that other area.

SECTION 8

Liabilities of Coroner. Removal and punishment of coroner

8. (1) The Lord Chancellor may, if he thinks fit, remove any coroner from his office for inability or misbehaviour in the discharge of his duty.

(2) A coroner who is guilty of extortion or of corruption or of wilful neglect of his duty or of misbehaviour in the discharge of his duty shall be guilty of a misdemeanor, and in addition to any other punishment may, unless his office of coroner is annexed to any other office, be adjudged by the court before whom he is so convicted to be removed from his office, and to be disqualified for acting as coroner, [...] and another coroner [shall be appointed in like manner] as in the case of any other vacancy.

COMMENTARY ON SECTION 8

Amendments

The words omitted in subsection 2 were repealed by the 1926 Act, s.31, Schedule 3.

The words in square brackets were inserted by the 1926 Act, s.30 and Schedule 2.

General Note

The Criminal Law Act 1967 abolished the distinction between misdemeanour and felony but made no reference to this section.

SECTION 9 [Repealed]

[9.]

SECTION 10 [Repealed]

[10.]

Note. Sections 9 and 10 were repealed by the Criminal Law Act 1977, s.65 and Schedule 13.

SECTION 11 [Abolished]

[11.]

Note. Section 11 was abolished by the Local Government Act 1888, s.5(6).

SECTION 12 [Repealed]

[12.]

Note. Section 12 was repealed by the 1926 Act, s.31 and Schedule 3. See now section 1 of that Act, *post,* at page 102.

SECTION 13 [Repealed]

[13.]

Note. Section 13 was repealed by the Coroners Act 1892, and Schedule. See now s.1 of that Act, *post,* at page 102.

SECTION 14 [Repealed]

[14.]

Note. Section 14 was repealed by the Local Government Act 1888, s.5(6).

SECTION 15 [Repealed]

[15.]

Note. Section 15 was repealed by the Courts Act 1971, s.56(4) and Schedule 11, Part IV.

SECTION 16 [Repealed]

[16.]

Note. Section 16 was repealed by the Criminal Law Act 1977, s.65 and Schedule 13.

SECTION 17

Prohibition on coroner taking fee

17. Save as is authorized by this or any other Act, a coroner shall not take any fee or remuneration in respect of anything done by him in the execution of his office.

COMMENTARY ON SECTION 17

"any fee or remuneration" in section 17. Fees for providing copies of documents are prescribed by the Coroners (Fees for Copies) Rules (currently S.I. 1982 No. 995) made under s.29(2)(*a*) of the 1926 Act.

PART II

SUPPLEMENTAL

SECTION 18

Enactments with respect to procedure at inquests

18. The following enactments shall be made with respect to procedure at coroners' inquests:

(1) The inquisition shall be under the hands [...] of the jurors who concur in the verdict, and of the coroner:

(2) An inquisition need not [...] be on parchment, and may be written or printed, or partly written and partly printed, and may be in the form contained in the Second Schedule to this Act, or to the like effect or in such other form as the Lord Chancellor from time to time prescribes, or to the like effect, and the statements therein may be made in concise and ordinary language.

(3) The coroner after the termination of an inquest on any death shall send to the registrar of deaths whose duty it is by law to register the death such certificate [...] and within such time as is required by the Registration Acts.

[(4).]
[(5).]
[(6).]

COMMENTARY ON SECTION 18

Amendments

In subsection (1) the words omitted were repealed by the 1926 Act, ss.30 and 31 and Schedules 2 and 3.

The words omitted in subsection (2) were repealed by the Indictments Act 1915, s.9 and Schedule 2.

The words omitted in subsection (3) were repealed by the 1926 Act, ss.30 and 31 and Schedules 2 and 3.

Subsections 4 and 5 were repealed by the Criminal Law Act 1977, s.65(5) and Schedule 13.

Subsection 6 was repealed by the 1926 Act, subsections 30 and 31 and Schedules 2 and 3.

General Note

"The inquisition." For the rules governing the obtaining of copies of depositions and the inquisition see S.I. 1982 No. 995.

See also the 1926 Act, s.20(5) as amended by the Criminal Law Act 1977, s.56 and Schedule 10.

For the appropriate Form of Inquisition see S.I. 1984 No. 552, Schedule 4, Form 22, *ante*, at page 72.

See also Rule 57 of the 1984 Rules (S.I. 1984 No. 552), *ante*, at page 59.

SECTION 19

Attendance of witnesses and jurors

19. (1) Where a person duly summoned as a juror at an inquest does not, after being openly called three times, appear to such summons, or appearing, refuses without reasonable excuse to serve as a juror, the coroner may impose on such person a fine not exceeding [two hundred pounds].

(2) Where a person duly summoned to give evidence at an inquest does not, after being openly called three times, appear to such summons, or appearing, refuses without lawful excuse to answer a question put to him, the coroner may impose on such person a fine not exceeding [two hundred pounds].

(3) Any power by this Act vested in a coroner of imposing a fine on a juror or witness, shall be deemed to be in addition to and not in derogation of any power the coroner may possess independently of this Act, for compelling any person to appear and give evidence before him on any inquest or other proceeding, or for punishing any person for contempt of court in not so appearing and giving evidence with this qualification, that a person shall not be fined by the coroner under this Act, and also be punished under the power of a coroner independently of this Act.

[(3a) Notwithstanding anything in the foregoing provisions of this section, no juror shall be liable to any penalty for non-attendance on a coroner's jury, unless the summons requiring him to attend was duly served on him no later than six days before the day on which he was required to attend.]

[(4)]

(5) Where a recognizance is forfeited at an inquest held before a coroner, the coroner shall proceed in like manner under this section as if he had

imposed a fine under this section upon the person forfeiting that recognizance, and the provisions of this section shall apply accordingly.

COMMENTARY ON SECTION 19

Amendments

In subsections (1) and (2) the words in square brackets were substituted by the Contempt of Court Act 1981, s.14 and Schedule 2, Part 3, paragraph 1.

Subsection (3a) was added by the Juries Act 1974, s.22(1) and Schedule 2.

Subsection (4) was repealed by the Criminal Justice Act 1967, s.103(2) and Schedule 7, Part 1.

General Note

"Does not ... appear to such summons ... " in Section 19(1). If a warrant is then issued, there is no power to execute the warrant outside the particular coroner's jurisdiction. A Crown Office subpoena may be required.

"Fine." The fines in subsections (1) and (2) and section 23, *post*, may be altered by order under the Magistrates' Courts Act 1980, s.143, as amended.

Contempt. The Coroners' Court is an inferior court of record, and has power to [fine] and commit for contempt (*Att. Gen.* v. *B.B.C.* [1981] A.C. 303; [1980] 3 All E.R. 161 considered): *R.* v. *West Yorkshire Coroner, ex parte Smith, The Times,* October 3, 1984, D.C. See also *Peart* v. *Stewart* [1983] A.C. 109; [1983] 1 All E.R. 859, H.L. The Contempt of Court Act 1981, s.14(1) permits an inferior court to commit a contemptor to prison for a maximum of one month. Section 14(2) of *ibid.* provides a ceiling of £500 in respect of powers to fine for a civil contempt in an inferior court.

SECTION 20 [Repealed]

[20.]

Note. Section 20 was repealed by the Criminal Law Act 1977, s.65 and Schedule 13.

SECTION 21

Medical Witnesses and Post-mortem Examinations. Power of coroner to summon medical witnesses and to direct performance of post-mortem examination

21. (1) Where it appears to the coroner that the deceased was attended at his death or during his last illness by any legally qualified medical practitioner, the coroner may summon such practitioner as a witness; but if it appears to the coroner that the deceased person was not attended at his death or during his last illness by any legally qualified medical practitioner, the coroner may summon any legally qualified medical practitioner who is at the time in actual practice in or near the place where the death happened, and any such medical witness as is summoned in pursuance of this section, may be asked to give evidence as to how, in his opinion, the deceased came to his death.

(2) The coroner may, either in his summons for the attendance of such medical witness or at any time between the issuing of that summons and the end of the inquest, direct such medical witness to make a post-mortem examination of the body of the deceased [. . .].

Provided that where a person states upon oath before the coroner that in his belief the death of the deceased was caused partly or entirely by the improper or negligent treatment of a medical practitioner or other person, such medical practitioner or other person shall not be allowed to perform or assist at the post-mortem examination of the deceased.

(3) If a majority of the jury sitting at an inquest are of opinion that the cause of death has not been satisfactorily explained by the evidence of the medical practitioner or other witnesses brought before them, they may require the coroner in writing to summon as a witness some other legally qualified medical practitioner named by them, and further to direct a post-mortem examination of the deceased [. . .], to be made by such last-mentioned practitioner, and that whether such examination has been previously made or not, and the coroner shall comply with such requisition, and in default shall be guilty of a misdemeanor.

COMMENTARY ON SECTION 21

Amendments

In subsection (2) the words omitted were repealed by the 1926 Act, s.30 and s.31 and Schedules 2 and 3.

In subsection (3) the words omitted were repealed by *ibid.*

General Note

Post-mortem examination. See S.I. 1984 No. 552, rules 5–11, *ante*, pages 39–42.

SECTION 22 [Repealed]

[22.]

Note. Section 22 was repealed by the 1926 Act, s.31 and Schedule 3.

SECTION 23

Penalty on medical practitioner for neglecting to attend

23. Where a medical practitioner fails to obey a summons of a coroner issued in pursuance of this Act, he shall, unless he shows a good and sufficient cause for not having obeyed the same, be liable on summary conviction on the prosecution of the coroner or of any two of the jury, to a fine not exceeding [two hundred pounds].

COMMENTARY ON SECTION 23

Amendments

The words in brackets were substituted by the Contempt of Court Act 1981, s.14(5) and Schedule 2, Part 3.

General Note

See Note to s.19, *ante*, at page 89.
The medical practitioner must be duly summoned for his non-attendance to be a contempt. *Re A. S. Rayan, The Times,* October 20, 1983.

SECTION 24 [Repealed]

[24.]

Note. Section 24 was repealed by the 1926 Act, s.31 and Schedule 3.

SECTION 25

Expenses and Returns of Inquests. Schedule of fees and disbursements payable on holding inquest

25. The local authority for a county [. . .] from time to time may make, and when made may alter and vary a schedule of fees, allowances, and disbursements which [. . .] may lawfully be paid and made by [a coroner in the course of his duties] [. . .], and the local authority shall cause a copy of every such schedule [. . .] to be delivered to every coroner concerned.

[**25A.**—(1) Subject to section 29(7A) below, a person who serves as a juror in a coroner's court shall be entitled, in respect of his attendance at court for the purpose of performing jury service, to receive payments, at [rates determined by the Secretary of State with the consent of the Minister for the Civil Service] and subject to any prescribed conditions, by way of allowance—

(*a*) for travelling and subsistence; and
(*b*) for financial loss where in consequence of his attendance for that purpose he has incurred any expenditure (otherwise than on travelling and subsistence) to which he would not otherwise be subject or he has suffered any loss of earnings, or of benefit under the enactments relating to national insurance and social security, which he would otherwise have made or received.

(2) The amount due to any person in respect of such service shall be ascertained and paid over to him by the coroner.

(3) In subsection (1) above the expression "prescribed" means prescribed by regulations made by statutory instrument by the Secretary of State with the consent of the Minister for the Civil Service; and for the purposes of that

91

subsection a person who, in obedience to a summons to serve on a jury, attends for service as a juror shall be deemed to serve as a juror notwithstanding that he is not subsequently sworn].

[(4).]

COMMENTARY ON SECTION 25

Amendments

The words omitted in the first and fifth set of square brackets were repealed by the Local Government Act 1972, s.220(5) and Schedule 30.

The words omitted in the second set of square brackets were repealed by the 1926 Act, s.31 and Schedule 3.

The words in the third set of square brackets were substituted by the 1926 Act, s.30 and Schedule 2.

The words omitted in the fourth set of square brackets were repealed by the Coroners Act 1954, s.1 and Schedule. See now s.1 of *ibid.* for fees and expenses of witnesses and medical practitioners, post at page 121.

Section 25A was added by the Juries Act 1974, s.22(1) and Schedule 2.

The words in square brackets in section 25A were substituted by the Administration of Justice Act 1977, s.2 and Schedule 2, paragraph 1.

Section 25A(4) was repealed by *ibid.*, s.32(4) and Schedule 5.

SECTION 26

Payment of expenses by coroner

26. A coroner holding an inquest shall immediately after the termination of the proceedings pay the fees of every medical witness [the allowances of every juror] [...] and all expenses reasonably incurred in and about the holding thereof, not exceeding the [fees, allowances and disbursements which may be lawfully paid or made under this Act and any fees, allowances, or disbursements so paid or made] shall be repaid to the coroner in manner provided by this Act.

COMMENTARY ON SECTION 26

Amendments

The words in the first set of square brackets were added by the Juries Act 1974, s.22(1) and Schedule 2.

The words in the third set of square brackets were substituted by the 1926 Act, s.30 and Schedule 2.

The words omitted in square brackets were repealed by the 1926 Act, s.31 and Schedule 3.

SECTION 27

Coroners to lay their accounts before the local authority

27. (1) Every coroner shall, within four months after [paying or making any fees, allowances or disbursements in accordance with the provisions of this Act, cause a full and true account of all fees, allowances and disbursements so paid or made] by him under this Act to be laid before the local authority of the county [...] by whom the sums are to be reimbursed to him.

(2) Every account shall be accompanied by such vouchers as under the circumstances may to the local authority seem reasonable, and the local authority may, if they think fit, examine the said coroner on oath as to the account, and on being satisfied of the correctness thereof, the local authority shall order their treasurer to pay to the coroner the sum due to him on such account, [...] and the treasurer shall pay the same out of the local rate, without any abatement or deduction whatever, and shall be allowed the same on passing his accounts.

COMMENTARY ON SECTION 27

Amendments

In subsection (1) the words in square brackets were substituted by the 1926 Act, s.30 and Schedule 2.

The words omitted in subsection (1) were repealed by the Local Government Act 1972, s.272(1) and Schedule 30.

The words omitted in subsection (2) were repealed by the 1926 Act, s.30 and Schedule 2.

SECTION 28

Coroners to make yearly returns to Secretary of State

28. Every coroner [...] shall on or before the first day of February in every year make and transmit to a Secretary of State a return in writing, in such form and containing such particulars as the Secretary of State from time to time directs, of all cases in which an inquest has been held by him, or by some person in lieu of him, during the year ending on the thirty-first day of December immediately preceding.

COMMENTARY ON SECTION 28

Amendments

The words omitted were repealed by the 1926 Act, s.31 Schedule 3.

SECTION 29

Coroner of the Queen's Household. Appointment and jurisdiction of the coroner of the Queen's household

29. (1) The coroner of Her Majesty the Queen's household shall continue to be appointed by the Lord Steward for the time being of the Queen's household.

(2) The coroner of the Queen's household shall have exclusive jurisdiction in respect of inquests on persons whose bodies are lying within the limits of any of the Queen's palaces or within the limits of any other house where Her Majesty is then demurrant and abiding in her own royal person, notwithstanding the subsequent removal of Her Majesty from such palace or house.

(3) The jurors on an inquest held by the coroner of the Queen's household shall consist of officers of the Queen's household, to be returned by such officer of the Queen's household as may be directed to summon the same by the warrant of the said coroner.

(4) The limits of the said palace or house shall be deemed to extend to any courts, gardens, or other places within the curtilage of such palace or house but not further, and where a body is lying dead in any place beyond those limits, the coroner of the Queen's household shall not have jurisdiction to hold an inquest on such [person], and the coroner of the county [. . .] shall have jurisdiction to hold that inquest in the same manner as if that place were not within the verge.

[(5).]

(6) All other inquisitions, depositions, and recognizances shall be delivered to the Lord Steward of the Queen's household to be filed among the records of his office.

(7) The coroner of the Queen's household shall make his declaration of office before the Lord Steward of the Queen's household, and shall reside in one of the Queen's palaces, or in such other convenient place as may from time to time be allowed by the Lord Steward of the Queen's household.

[(7A) Section 25A of this Act shall not apply in relation to service on a jury under this section but that shall not affect any entitlement to payment that may otherwise be enjoyed by a juror for service on such a jury.]

(8) Save as is in this section specially provided, the coroner of the Queen's household shall, within the said limits have the same jurisdiction and powers, be subject to the same obligations, liabilities, and disqualifications, and generally to the provisions of this Act and to the law relating to coroners in like manner as any other franchise coroner.

[(9).]

COMMENTARY ON SECTION 29

Amendments

In subsection (4) the word in square brackets was substituted by the Coroners Act 1980, Schedule 1, para 2.

The words omitted in subsection (4) were repealed by the Local Government Act 1972 (c. 70), s.272(1) and Schedule 30.

Subsections (5) and (9) were repealed by the Criminal Law Act 1967 (c. 58), Schedule 3, Part III.

Subsection (7A) was added by the Juries Act 1974, s.22(1) and Schedule 2.

SECTION 30 [Repealed]

[30.]

SECTION 31 [Repealed]

[31.]

SECTION 32 [Repealed]

[32.]

SECTION 33 [Repealed]

[33.]

Note. Sections 30–33 were repealed by the Local Government Act 1972, s.272(1) and Schedule 30.

SECTION 34

Saving clause as to official coroners

34. Nothing in this Act shall prejudice the jurisdiction of a judge exercising the jurisdiction of a coroner by virtue of his office, and such judge may, notwithstanding the passing of this Act, exercise any jurisdiction, statutable or otherwise, previously exercisable by him, in the same manner as if this Act had not passed.

COMMENTARY ON SECTION 34

General Note

"Jurisdiction of a judge." The Lord Chief Justice and all High Court judges are *ex officio* coroners. See Halsbury's *Laws of England*, Vol. 9 (4th edn.), par. 1004.

SECTION 35

Saving of jurisdiction as to removal of coroner, or otherwise in relation to a coroner

35. Nothing in this Act shall prejudice the jurisdiction of the Lord Chancellor or the High Court [. . .] in relation to removing a coroner otherwise than in manner provided by this Act, or in any manner prejudice or affect the jurisdiction of the High Court [. . .] or of any judge thereof in relation to or over a coroner or his duties.

COMMENTARY ON SECTION 35

Amendments

The words omitted were repealed by the Statute Law Revision Act 1908.

SECTION 36

Inquest on treasure trove

36. A coroner shall continue as heretofore to have jurisdiction to inquire of treasure that is found, who were the finders, and who is suspected thereof, and the provisions of this Act shall, so far as is consistent with the tenor thereof, apply to every such inquest.

COMMENTARY ON SECTION 36

General Note

"treasure trove" is any gold or silver in coin, plate, or bullion found concealed in a house, or in the earth or other private place, the owner thereof being unknown; the treasure belongs to the Queen or her grantee having the franchise of treasure trove: *A.G.* v. *Moore* [1893] 1 Ch. 676 at p. 683, *per* Stirling J.

"treasure." The Crown's right to treasure trove is limited to articles (including coins) of gold and silver. Whether an object is silver is a question of fact for the jury: *A.G. of the Duchy of Lancaster* v. *G.E. Overton (Farms) Ltd.* [1982] 2 W.L.R. 397, C.A., [1982] 1 All E.R. 524.

The coroner is confined to determining "who was the finder and who is suspected thereof." He has no power to inquire into the question of title: *A. G.* v. *Moore* [1893] 1 Ch. 676.

Although the 1887 Act applies to inquests on treasure trove "so far as is consistent with the tenor thereof," *e.g.* number of jurors, the 1984 Coroners Rules do not apply; see rule 2(1) (where inquest for the purpose of these rules is defined as meaning an inquest for the purpose of inquiring into the death of a person).

Procedure. It is the coroner's duty, as soon as the finding of any treasure becomes known to him, to summon a jury and inquire into the facts. The coroner hears the evidence and he directs the jury as to the meaning of treasure trove. He will then usually put the following questions to the jury: of what did the find consist; where was it deposited; was it intentionally hidden or concealed, or accidentally lost, or purposely abandoned (to be treasure trove it must have been intentionally hidden); is the owner unknown (the owner must be unknown if the find is to be treasure trove); who was the finder (he may be rewarded); did the finder conceal his find. If the answers given by the jury to these questions indicate the find to be treasure trove, the coroner will declare it to be so.

SECTION 37

Effect of Schedules

37. The Schedules to this Act shall be construed and have effect as part of this Act, and the forms given in any of those schedules, or such other forms as the Lord Chancellor from time to time directs, may be used in all matters to which they apply, and when so used shall be sufficient in law.

SECTION 38 [Repealed]

[38.]

SECTION 39 [Repealed]

[39.]

SECTION 40 [Repealed]

[40.]

Note. Sections 38–40 were repealed by the Local Government Act 1972, s.272(1) and Schedule 30.

SECTION 41

Definition of "local authority" and "local rate"

41. For the purposes of this Act—

[(*a*)]
[(*b*)]
  (*c*) the local rate shall be [. . .] the county rate [. . .].
[(*d*)].

COMMENTARY ON SECTION 41

Amendments

Subsections (*a*) and (*b*) were repealed by the Local Government Act 1972, s.272(1) and Schedule 30.
  The words omitted in subsection (*c*) were repealed by *ibid.*
  Subsection (*d*) was repealed by the Statute Law Revision Act 1908.

SECTION 42

Definitions. "Franchise coroner"

42. In this Act, if not inconsistent with the context, the following terms and expressions have the meanings hereinafter respectively assigned to them:

[...]

The expression "franchise coroner" means any of the following coroners, that is to say, the coroner of the Queen's household, [a coroner or deputy coroner for the jurisdiction of the Admiralty, a coroner appointed by Her Majesty the Queen in right of Her Duchy of Lancaster, and a coroner appointed for a town corporate, liberty, lordship, manor, university, or other place, the coroner for which has heretofore been appointed by any lord, or otherwise than by election of the freeholders of a county, or of any part of a county, or by the council of a borough, and the expression "franchise" means the area within which the franchise coroner exercises jurisdiction].

[...]

The expression "Registration Acts" means the Acts for the time being in force relating to the registration of deaths, inclusive of any enactment amending the same.

COMMENTARY ON SECTION 42

Amendments

The words omitted in the first set of square brackets were repealed by the Statute Law Revision Act 1908.

The words in square brackets were made otiose by the Local Government Act 1972, but were not specifically repealed by it.

The words omitted in the third set of square brackets were repealed by the Statute Law Revision Act 1908 and the Criminal Law Act 1967, Schedule 3.

General Note

Although not completely repealed, many of the types of coroner mentioned in section 42 no longer exist. Franchise coroners (except the coroner for the Queen's Household) were abolished by section 220(1) of the Local Government Act 1972.

SECTION 43

Temporary Provisions and Repeal. Saving as to coroners' salaries and districts

43. Nothing in this Act shall affect the law respecting the salaries of coroners for counties, or the division of a county into coroners' districts, or the rights and duties of coroners as respects such districts.

SECTION 44 [Repealed].

[44.]

Note. Section 44 was repealed by the Criminal Law Act 1967, s.10(2) and Schedule 3, Part 1.

SECTION 45

Repeal of Acts in schedule

45. The Acts specified in the Third Schedule to this Act are hereby repealed, from and after the passing of this Act, to the extent specified in the third column of that schedule.

Provided that—

[(1.)]

(2) Any schedule of fees, allowances, and disbursements made by a local authority for a county or borough before the passing of this Act shall, until a schedule is made in pursuance of this Act, be of the same effect as if the schedule had been made in pursuance of this Act, and

[(3.)]

[(4.)]

(5) Save in so far as is inconsistent with this Act, any principle or rule of law, or established jurisdiction, practice, or procedure, or existing usage, franchise, liberty, or custom, shall, notwithstanding the repeal of any enactment by this Act, remain in full force.

COMMENTARY ON SECTION 45

Amendments

Paragraphs 1, 3 and 4 of the proviso were repealed by the Statute Law Revision Act 1908.

THE CORONERS ACT 1892

(55 & 56 Vict. c. 56)

An Act to amend the Law in relation to the Appointment of Coroners and Deputy Coroners in Counties and Boroughs.

[28th June 1892.]

BE it enacted by the Queen's most Excellent Majesty, by and with the advice and consent of the Lords Spiritual and Temporal, and Commons, in this present Parliament assembled, and by the authority of the same, as follows:

SECTION 1

Appointment and powers of a deputy coroner of both a county and a borough

1.—(1) Every coroner [...] shall appoint, by writing under his hand, a fit person approved by the chairman [...] of the council who appointed the coroner, [...] to be his deputy, and may revoke such appointment, but such revocation shall not take effect until the appointment of another deputy has been approved as aforesaid.

(2) A duplicate of every appointment shall be sent to the said council and be kept among the records of the county [...]

(3) A deputy may act for the coroner during his illness or during his absence for any lawful or reasonable cause, or at any inquest which the coroner is disqualified for holding, but not otherwise. [...]

(4) The deputy of a coroner shall, notwithstanding the coroner vacates his office by death or otherwise, continue in office until a new deputy is appointed, and shall act as the coroner while the office is so vacant in like manner as during the illness of the coroner, [...] and he shall be entitled to receive in respect of the period of the vacancy the like remuneration as the vacating coroner.

(5) For the purpose of an inquest or act which a deputy of a coroner is authorised to hold or do, he shall be deemed to be that coroner, and have the same jurisdiction and powers and be subject to the same obligations, liabilities, and disqualifications as that coroner, and he shall generally be subject to the provisions of the Coroners Act, 1887, and to the law relating to coroners in like manner as that coroner.

(6) A council may postpone the appointment of a coroner to fill a vacancy, either generally or in any particular case, for a period not exceeding three months from the date at which that vacancy occurs.

[(7).]

(8) In the case of a county coroner who has been elected before the date on which the provisions of the Local Government Act, 1888, as to the appointment of coroners came into force, the council of any county or county borough, in which the district of the coroner is wholly or partially situated, shall for the purposes of this section be deemed to be the council who appointed the coroner.

COMMENTARY ON SECTION 1

Amendments

The words omitted in the first and second square brackets in subsection (1) and in the square brackets in subsection (2) were repealed by the Local Government Act, 1972, s.272(1) and Schedule 30.

The words omitted in the third set of square brackets in subsection (1) were repealed by the Coroners (Amendment) Act, 1926, s.31 and Schedule 3.

The words omitted in subsections (3) and (4) were repealed by *ibid.*

Subsection (7) was repealed by the Local Government Act 1972, s.272(1) and Schedule 30.

SECTION 2

Repeal

2. The Acts specified in the schedule to this Act are hereby repealed to the extent in the third column of that schedule mentioned.

SECTION 3

Construction of Act and short title

3. This Act shall be construed as one with the Coroners Act 1887, and this Act and that Act may be cited together as the Coroners Acts, 1887 and 1892, and this Act may be cited separately as the Coroners Act, 1892.

SCHEDULE

Session and Chapter.	Short Title.	Extent of Repeal.
45 & 46 Vict. c. 50.	The Municipal Corporations Act, 1882.	Section one hundred and seventy-two.
50 & 51 Vict. c. 71.	The Coroners Act, 1887.	Section thirteen, and in section thirty-three the words "and the "appointment of a "deputy by such "coroner."

THE CORONERS (AMENDMENT) ACT 1926

(16 & 17 Geo. 5, c. 59)

An Act to amend the law relating to coroners.

[December 15, 1926]

SECTION 1

Qualification, appointment, and resignation of coroners

1. (1) From and after the commencement of this Act no person shall be qualified to be appointed to be a coroner for a county (in this Act referred to as "a county coroner") [...] or a deputy or assistant deputy to a county [...] coroner, unless he is a barrister, solicitor, or legally qualified medical practitioner, of not less than five years standing in his profession.

[...]

(2) A person shall, so long as he [...] is alderman or councillor of a county [...] and for six months after he ceases to be [...] alderman or councillor thereof, be disqualified for being a coroner appointed by the council of that county [...] and for being a deputy of a coroner so appointed.

(3) A person shall, so long as he is a coroner for a county [...] or a deputy of such coroner, be disqualified for being a mayor, alderman or councillor of that county [...].

[(4).]

COMMENTARY ON SECTION 1

Amendments

The words omitted in subsection (1) were repealed by the Local Government Act 1972, s.272(1) and Schedule 30.

The words omitted in subsection (2) were repealed by *ibid.*

The words omitted in subsection (3) were repealed by *ibid.*

Subsection (4) was repealed by the Statute Law Revision Act 1950.

SECTION 2

Appointment and Resignation of county coroners

2. (1) On a vacancy occurring in the office of coroner for a county [...], the council having power to appoint a person to fill the vacancy shall forthwith give notice thereof to the Secretary of State.

(2) Subject to the provisions of this Act relating to the formation and alteration of coroners' districts, within three months after the occurrence of a vacancy in the office of coroner for a county [...] or within such further time as the Secretary of State may allow, the council having power to appoint a coroner shall appoint a duly qualified person to the office and shall forthwith give notice of the appointment to the Secretary of State.

(3) A county [...] coroner may resign his office by giving notice in writing to the council having power to appoint his successor, but the resignation shall not take effect unless and until it is accepted by the council.

(4) It shall not be necessary to issue a writ *de coronatore eligendo* or a writ *de coronatore exonerando* in respect of the appointment or resignation of a county or borough coroner.

(5) Nothing in this section shall prejudice or affect the jurisdiction of the Lord Chancellor or of any court with respect to the removal of coroners.

COMMENTARY ON SECTION 2

Amendments

The words omitted were repealed by The Local Government Act 1972 (c. 70), s.272(1) and Schedule 30.

SECTION 3 [Repealed]

[3.]

SECTION 4 [Repealed]

[4.]

Note. Sections 3 and 4 were repealed by the Local Government Act 1972, s.272(1) and Schedule 30.

SECTION 5

Salaries and pensions of county coroners

5. (1) Subject to the provisions of this section every council having power to appoint a coroner shall pay to every county [...] coroner appointed by them an annual salary at such rate as may be fixed by agreement between them and the coroner.

(2) If at any time a coroner and the council by whom his salary is payable are unable to agree with respect to any proposed alteration of the rate of salary, the Secretary of State may, upon the application either of the coroner or of the council, fix the rate of the salary at such rate as he thinks proper, and thereupon the rate so fixed by the Secretary of State shall come into force as from such date as he may determine, not being a date less than three years from the date when the rate of salary came into force as last fixed,

unless in the opinion of the Secretary of State the coroner's area or district has in the meantime been materially altered.

(3) In fixing the rate of salary payable to a coroner under this section regard shall be had to the nature and extent of his duties and to all the circumstances of the case.

[(4).]

(5) As respects coroners holding office at the commencement of this Act—

(a) every coroner to whom a salary is, at the commencement of this Act, payable by the council of any county shall for the purposes of this section be deemed to have been appointed by that council and to be a county coroner; and

(b) the salary of a county coroner shall, subject to any alteration which may subsequently be made under this section, continue to be payable at the rate in force at the commencement of this Act; and

(c) the salary of a borough coroner shall in default of agreement between him and the council by whom his salary is payable be at a rate fixed by the Secretary of State.

COMMENTARY ON SECTION 5

The words omitted in subsection (1) were repealed by The Local Government Act 1972, s.272(1) and Schedule 30.

Subsection (4) was repealed by *ibid*.

SECTION 6

Superannuation of county coroners

6. (1) Upon the retirement of any county [. . .] coroner after not less than five years service, the council by whom his salary is payable shall have power—

(a) if he has attained the age of sixty-five years; or

(b) if they are satisfied by means of a medical certificate that he is incapable from infirmity of mind or body of discharging the duties of his office, and that such incapacity is likely to be permanent

to grant to him a pension of such amount as may be agreed upon between him and the council not exceeding the scale contained in the First Schedule to this Act:

Provided that the provisions of this section shall not apply with respect to any coroner holding office at the date of the commencement of this Act unless upon his application a resolution applying those provisions to him is passed by the council by whom his salary is payable.

(2) A county [. . .] coroner with respect to whom the provisions of this section apply shall at any time after he has completed fifteen years service and has attained the age of sixty-five years, vacate his office if called upon to do so by the council by whom his salary is payable, but shall, in the absence of agreement to the contrary, in that case be entitled to receive the maximum pension which the council is empowered having regard to the length of his service to grant to him under this section.

(3) For the purposes of this section the expression "service" means service, whether before or after the commencement of this Act, as a coroner in the county [. . .] of the council by whom the pension is payable.

COMMENTARY ON SECTION 6

Amendments

The words omitted in square brackets were repealed by The Local Government Act 1972, s.272(1) and Schedule 30.

General Note

Subsection (1) and Schedule 1 (pensions for coroners) were disapplied in respect of coroners:

(a) appointed on or after 6 April 1978; or
(b) holding office as coroner immediately before 6 April 1978 and electing in writing before 6 July 1978 that the provisions of the 1926 Act relating to pensions shall not apply to him from 6 July 1978.

(Social Security (Modification of Coroners (Amendment) Act 1926) Order 1978 (S.I. 1978 No. 374))
See also the Local Government Superannuation (Amendment) (No. 2) Regulations 1978 (S.I. 1978 No. 822).

SECTION 7

Payment of salaries and pensions

7. The salary of a county [. . .] coroner and any pension payable to a person in respect of his service as a coroner, shall be deemed to accrue from day to day, and, in the absence of agreement to the contrary, shall be payable quarterly.

COMMENTARY ON SECTION 7

Amendments

The words omitted in section 7 were repealed by The Local Government Act 1972, s.272(1) and Schedule 30.

SECTION 8 [Repealed]

[8.]

Note. Section 8 was repealed by *ibid.* and section 220(5) of *ibid.*

SECTION 9 [Repealed]

[9.]

Note. Section 9 was repealed by the Statute Law Revision Act 1950.

SECTION 10

Appointment of deputy by coroner of King's household

10. The Coroners Act, 1892 (which relates to the appointment and powers of deputy coroners) shall apply with the necessary modifications to the coroner of the King's household as it applies to county [...] coroners, and in particular with the modifications that the appointment of a deputy to the coroner of the King's household shall be subject to the approval of the Lord Steward of the King's household, and duplicates of such appointments shall be sent to and kept by him.

COMMENTARY ON SECTION 10

Amendments

The words omitted in section 10 were repealed by the Local Government Act 1972, s.272(1) and Schedule 30.

SECTION 11

Appointment of assistant deputy coroner

11.—(1) Any county [...] coroner may, in addition to the deputy whom he is required to appoint under section one of the Coroners Act, 1892, appoint an assistant deputy to act for the coroner.

(2) An assistant deputy may act for the coroner on any occasion when the deputy coroner would be entitled to act for the coroner but is unable so to act owing to illness or absence for any reasonable cause, and, in the event of the coroner vacating his office by death or otherwise, may act for the deputy coroner in like manner while the office of coroner is vacant.

(3) The appointment of an assistant deputy shall be made in the like manner and subject to the like approval as the appointment of a deputy coroner, and shall be revocable at any time by the coroner by writing under his hand: duplicates of any such appointment or revocation shall be sent to and preserved by the council who appointed the coroner in like manner as duplicates of the appointment of a deputy coroner.

(4) Subsection (5) of the said section one of the Coroners Act, 1892, shall apply as respects any inquest or act which an assistant deputy of a coroner is authorized to hold or do, with the substitution of a reference to an assistant deputy for the reference to a deputy.

COMMENTARY ON SECTION 11

Amendments

The words omitted in subsection (1) were repealed by the Local Government Act 1972, s.272(1) and Schedule 30.

SECTION 12

Coroners' Districts: Formation and alteration of county coroners' districts

12.—(1) A county council may at any time, and shall if directed to do so by the Secretary of State, submit, after complying with such requirements as to notice and consideration of objections as may be prescribed, to the Secretary of State a draft order providing for the division of the county into such coroners' districts as they think expedient, or for such alteration of any existing division of the county into coroners' districts as appears to them to be suitable; and the Secretary of State after taking into consideration any objections to the draft made in the prescribed manner and within the prescribed time, may make the order, either in the terms of the draft submitted to him or with such modifications as he thinks fit.

(2) Every order made under this section shall come into force as from such date as may be specified in the order, and may be varied or revoked by any subsequent order made in like manner.

(3) If by reason of any order made under this section it is in the opinion of the Secretary of State necessary that the number of coroners for a county should be increased, the county council shall appoint such number of additional coroners for the county as the Secretary of State may direct, and the provisions of this Act relating to appointments to the office of county coroner shall apply with respect to any such appointment as if a vacancy had occurred in the office of coroner for that county.

(4) Sections five, nineteen and twenty of the Coroners Act, 1844 (which relate to the assignment of districts to county coroners and to the [...] jurisdiction of county coroners within counties assigned to them) shall, as amended by any subsequent enactment, apply to districts formed or altered and to coroners appointed under this Act as they apply to districts formed under that Act and to coroners appointed under writs *de coronatore eligendo*.

(5) Every order made under this section shall be laid as soon as may be before both Houses of Parliament and shall be published in the London Gazette, and particulars of any order so made shall be published by the county council in such manner as may be prescribed.

(6) Section one of the Rules Publication Act, 1893, shall not apply to any order made under this section.

(7) In this section the expression "prescribed" means prescribed by the Secretary of State either by general rules or by directions given as respects any particular occasion.

COMMENTARY ON SECTION 12

Amendments

The words omitted in subsection (4) were repealed by the Local Government Act 1972, s.272(1) and Schedule 30.

General Note

By virtue of the Local Government Act 1972, s.220(3), section 12 of the 1926 Act does not apply in relation to the City and Temples to which the Coroners Acts otherwise apply "as if together they were a county and the Common Council were the council of that County."

INQUESTS

SECTION 13

Power to hold inquest without a jury in certain cases

13.—(1) Subject to the provisions of this section, a coroner within whose jurisdiction the dead body of a person is lying, may, in lieu of summoning a jury in the manner required by section three of the Coroners Act, 1887, for the purpose of inquiring into the death of that person, hold an inquest [into the death of that person] without a jury.

(2) If it appears to the coroner either before he proceeds to hold an inquest or in the course of an inquest begun without a jury, that there is reason to suspect—

    [(*a*)]

    (*b*) that the death occurred in prison or in such place or in such circumstances as to require an inquest under any Act other than the Coroners Act, 1887; or

    (*c*) that the death was caused by an accident, poisoning or disease notice of which is required to be given to a government department, or to any inspector or other officer of a government department, under or in pursuance of any Act, [or to an inspector appointed under s.19 of the Health and Safety at Work Act etc. 1974].

[(*d*)]
(*e*) that the death occurred in circumstances the continuance or possible recurrence of which is prejudicial to the health or safety of the public or any section of the public;
[(*f*) that the death occurred while the deceased was in police custody, or resulted from an injury caused by a police officer in the purported execution of his duty;]

he shall proceed to summon a jury in the manner required by the Coroners Act, 1887, and in any other case, if·it appears to him, either before he proceeds to hold an inquest or in the course of an inquest begun without a jury, that there is any reason for summoning a jury, he may proceed to summon a jury in the manner aforesaid.

(3) The provisions of any enactment relating to the procedure in connection with an inquest shall, as respects an inquest or any part of an inquest which is held without a jury, have effect subject to such modifications as are rendered necessary by the absence of a jury, and where the whole of an inquest is held without a jury the inquisition shall be under the hand of the coroner alone.

(4) Where an inquest or any part of an inquest is held without a jury, anything done at the inquest, or at that part of the inquest, by or before the coroner alone shall be as validly done as if it had been done by or before the coroner and a jury.

COMMENTARY ON SECTION 13

Amendments

In subsection (1) the words in square brackets were substituted by the Coroners Act 1980, s.1 and Schedule 1, paragraph 3.

Subsection (2) (*a*) and (*d*) were repealed by the Criminal Law Act 1977, s.56(2), 65 and Schedule 13.

In subsection (2) (*c*) the words in square brackets were added by the Health and Safety at Work etc. Act 1974, s.83 and Schedule 9.

Subsection 2 (*f*) was added by the Administration of Justice Act 1982, s.62.

General Note

Subsection 2 (*e*). A coroner must summon a jury when the circumstances of death are such that similar fatalities might recur and it is reasonable to expect that appropriate action by a responsible authority ought to be taken to prevent such recurrence: *R.* v. *Hammersmith Coroner, ex parte Peach,* [1980] Q.B. 211; [1980] 2 All E.R. 7, C.A.

For the Form of Inquisition at both jury and non-jury inquests see S.I. 1984 (No. 552, Schedule 4, Form 22 *ante*, at page 72.

"Where . . . any part of an inquest is held without a jury" in subsection 4. In *R.* v. *Surrey Coroner, ex parte Campbell, D.C.* [1982] Q.B. 661 it was held that although the coroner had heard the first part of the inquest without a jury and had come to a conclusion about the cause of death, the coroner had properly recalled the medical evidence for the benefit of the jury and, therefore, the provisions of section 13(4) were no longer applicable to continue to validate the coroner's prior decision as to the cause of death.

SECTION 14 [Repealed]

[14.]

Note. Section 14 was repealed by the Coroners Act 1980, s.1 and Schedule 2.

SECTION 15

Failure of jury to agree

15.—(1) If the jury at an inquest fails to agree on a verdict, and the minority consists of not more than two, the coroner may accept the verdict of the majority, and the majority shall, in that case, certify the verdict in accordance with the requirements of subsection (3) of section four of the Coroners Act, 1887.

(2) In any other case of disagreement the coroner may discharge the jury and issue a warrant for summoning another jury, and thereupon the inquest shall proceed in all respects as if the proceedings which terminated in the disagreement had not taken place [. . .].

COMMENTARY ON SECTION 15

Amendments

In subsection (2) the words omitted were repealed by the Coroners Act 1980, s.1 and Schedule 2.

SECTION 16 [Repealed]

[16.]

SECTION 17 [Repealed]

[17.]

Note. Sections 16 and 17 were repealed by The Coroners Act 1980, s.1 and Schedule 2 and are superseded by s.2 of *ibid.*

SECTION 18

Inquest where body destroyed or irrecoverable

18. Where a coroner has reason to believe that a death has occurred in or near the area within which he has jurisdiction in such circumstances that an inquest ought to be held, and that owing to the destruction of the body by fire or otherwise or to the fact that the body is lying in a place from which it cannot be recovered, an inquest cannot be held except by virtue of the provisions of this section, he may report the facts to the Secretary of State, and the Secretary of State may, if he considers it desirable so to do, direct an inquest to be held touching the death, and an inquest shall be held accordingly by the coroner making the report or such other coroner as the Secretary of State may direct, and the law relating to coroners and coroners' inquests shall apply with such modifications as may be necessary in consequence of the inquest being [one into the death of a person whose body does not lie] within the coroner's jurisdiction.

COMMENTARY ON SECTION 18

Amendments

In section 18 the words in square brackets were substituted by The Coroners Act 1980, s.1 and Schedule 1, paragraph 4.

General Note

It is a matter for the coroner whether or not to hold a section 18 inquest with a jury. Whether or not a jury should be summoned will be decided by the coroner in the normal way, *i.e.* does the death fall under any of the categories set out in, s.13 of the 1926 Act, *ante.* In most cases the coroner's reason for wishing to hold the inquest will fall under s.13(c)—that the death occurred in circumstances the continuance or possible recurrence of which is prejudicial to the health or safety of the public or any section of it—and will therefore require a jury.

SECTION 19

Effect of the Coroners Act 1887, s.6

19. For the removal of doubts it is hereby declared, without prejudice to the generality of the provisions of section six of the Coroners Act 1887, that the powers of the High Court under that section extend to and may be exercised in any case where the Court is satisfied that by reason of the discovery of new facts or evidence it is necessary or desirable in the interests of justice that an inquisition on an inquest previously held concerning a death should be quashed, and that another inquest should be held.

COMMENTARY ON SECTION 19

General Note

"by reason of the discovery of new facts or evidence . . ." See *R. v. Huntbach, ex parte Lockley* [1944] K.B. 606; [1944] 2 All E.R. 453.

SECTION 20

Amendments with respect to inquests in cases of murder, manslaughter or infanticide

[**20.**—(1) If on an inquest touching a death the coroner before the conclusion of the inquest—

(a) is informed by the clerk of a magistrates' court in pursuance of subs. (8) below that some person has been charged before a magistrates' court with—

(i) the murder, manslaughter or infanticide of the deceased; or

(ii) an offence under s.1 of the Road Traffic Act 1972 committed by causing the death of the deceased; or

(iii) an offence under s.2(1) of the Suicide Act 1961 consisting of aiding, abetting, counselling or procuring the suicide of the deceased; or

(b) is informed by the Director of Public Prosecutions that some person has been charged before examining justices with an offence (whether or not involving the death of a person other than the deceased) alleged to have been committed in circumstances connected with the death of the deceased, not being an offence within para. (a)(i), (ii) or (iii) above, and is requested by the Director to adjourn the inquest,

then, subject to subs. (2) below, the coroner shall, in the absence of reason to the contrary, adjourn the inquest until after the conclusion of the relevant criminal proceedings and, if a jury has been summoned, may, if he thinks fit, discharge them.

(2) The coroner—

(a) need not adjourn the inquest in a case within subs. (1) (a) above if, before he has done so, the Director of Public Prosecutions notifies him that adjournment is unnecessary; and

(b) may in any case resume the adjourned inquest before the conclusion of the relevant criminal proceedings if notified by the Director that it is open to him to do so.

(3) After the conclusion of the relevant criminal proceedings, or on being notified as mentioned in subs. (2)(b) above before their conclusion, the coroner may, subject to the following provisions of this section, resume the adjourned inquest if in his opinion there is sufficient cause to do so.

(4) Where a coroner adjourns an inquest in compliance with subs. (1) above, he shall furnish the registrar of deaths with a certificate under his hand stating the particulars which under the Births and Deaths Registration Act 1953 are required to be registered concerning the death, so far as they

have been ascertained at the date of the certificate; and the registrar shall enter the death and particulars in the form and manner prescribed by regulations under that Act.

(5) Where a coroner does not resume an inquest which he has adjourned in compliance with subs. (1) above, he shall (without prejudice to subs. (4) above) furnish the registrar of deaths with a certificate under his hand stating the result of the relevant criminal proceedings.

(6) Where a coroner resumes an inquest which has been adjourned in compliance with subs. (1) above and for that purpose summons a jury (but not where he resumes without a jury, or with the same jury as before the adjournment), he shall proceed in all respects as if the inquest had not previously been begun, and, subject to subs. (7) below, the provisions of this Act shall apply accordingly as if the resumed inquest were a fresh inquest [...].

(7) Where a coroner resumes an inquest which has been adjourned in compliance with subs. (1) above—

    (a) the finding of the inquest as to the cause of death must not be inconsistent with the outcome of the relevant criminal proceedings;

    (b) the coroner shall, after the termination of the inquest, furnish the registrar of deaths with a certificate under his hand stating the result of the relevant criminal proceedings; and

    (c) the provisions of para. (3) of s.18 of the Coroners Act 1887 and s.23(1) of the Births and Deaths Registration Act 1953 (duty of coroner to send registrar certificate containing information as to death and finding of inquest) shall not apply in relation to that inquest.

(8) Where a person is charged before a magistrates' court with murder, manslaughter or infanticide or an offence under s.1 of the Road Traffic Act 1972 (causing death by reckless driving) or an offence under s.2(1) of the Suicide Act 1961 consisting of aiding, abetting, counselling or procuring the suicide of another, the clerk of the court shall inform the coroner who is responsible for holding an inquest [touching the death] of the making of the charge and of the result of the proceedings before that court.

(9) Where a person charged with murder, manslaughter or infanticide or an offence under s.1 of the Road Traffic Act 1972 (causing death by reckless driving) or an offence under s.2(1) of the Suicide Act 1961 consisting of aiding, abetting, counselling or procuring the suicide of another, is committed for trial to the Crown Court, the appropriate officer of the Crown Court at the place where the person charged is tried shall inform the coroner of the result of the proceedings before that court.

(10) Where the Director of Public Prosecutions has in pursuance of paragraph (b) of subs. (1) above requested a coroner to adjourn an inquest, then, whether or not the inquest is adjourned as a result, the Director shall

inform the coroner of the result of the proceedings before the magistrates' court in the case of the person charged as mentioned in that paragraph and, if that person is committed for trial to the Crown Court, shall inform the coroner of the result of the proceedings before that court.

(11) In this section "the relevant criminal proceedings" means the proceedings before examining justices and before any court to which the person charged is committed for trial.]

COMMENTARY ON SECTION 20

Amendments

The new section 20 was substituted by the Criminal Law Act 1977, s.56(3) and Schedule 10.

In subsection (6) the words omitted were repealed by the Coroners Act 1980, s.1 and Schedule 1, paragraph 5.

In subsection (8) the words in square brackets were substituted by the Coroners Act 1980, s.1 and Schedule 1, paragraph 5.

General Note

For the rules governing adjournments see S.I. 1984 No. 552, Rules 25–35, *ante*. A coroner also has a general authority under his common law powers to adjourn an inquest for any reasonable cause if he thinks fit.

An inquest should not be adjourned *sine die* but rather to a specific date unless there is express or implied statutory authority to the contrary. (Inquests adjourned under s.7 of the visiting Forces Act 1952 *are* normally adjourned *sine die* since there is no intention of resuming them.) An inquest which is adjourned to a specific date but not resumed to a later date may be quashed on the ground that the inquest ended when the adjourned inquest was not resumed. See *R*. v. *Payn* (1864) 34 L.J.Q.B. 59; *R*. v. *Coroner for Margate* (1865) 10 Cox C.C. 64.

SECTION 21

Post-mortem and special examinations, without inquest

21. (1) Where a coroner is informed that the dead body of a person is lying within his jurisdiction and there is reasonable cause to suspect that the person has died a sudden death of which the cause is unknown, if the coroner is of opinion that a post-mortem examination may prove an inquest to be unnecessary he may direct any legally qualified medical practitioner whom, if an inquest were held, he would be entitled under section twenty-one of the Coroners Act, 1887, to summon as a medical witness or may request any other legally qualified medical practitioner, to make a post-mortem examination of the body of the deceased and to report the result thereof to him in writing, and for the purposes of the examination the coroner and any person directed or requested by him to make the examination shall have the like powers, authorities and immunities as if the

114

examination were a post-mortem examination directed by the coroner at an inquest [touching the death] of the deceased.

[(2).]

(3) Nothing in this section shall be construed as authorizing the coroner to dispense with an inquest in any case where there is reasonable cause to suspect that the deceased has died either a violent or an unnatural death, or has died in prison, or in such place or in such circumstances as to necessitate the holding of an inquest in accordance with the requirements of any Act other than the Coroners Act, 1887.

COMMENTARY ON SECTION 21

Amendments

In subsection (1) the words in square brackets were substituted by the Coroners Act 1980, s.1 and Schedule 1, paragraph 16.

Subsection (2) was repealed by the Births and Deaths Registration Act 1953, s.43(2) and Schedule 2. It was replaced by section 23(3) of *ibid.*

SECTION 22

Power of coroner to request specially qualified persons to make post-mortem and special examinations

22.—(1) Without prejudice to the power of a coroner holding an inquest to direct a medical witness whom he may summon under section twenty-one of the Coroners Act, 1887, to make a post-mortem examination of the body of the deceased, the coroner may, at any time after he has decided to hold an inquest, request any legally qualified medical practitioner to make—

(*a*) a post-mortem examination of the body of the deceased; or

(*b*) a special examination by way of analysis, test or otherwise of such parts or contents of the body or such other substances or things as ought in the opinion of the coroner to be submitted to analyses, tests or other special examination with a view to ascertaining how the deceased came by his death;

or to make both such examinations, or may request any person whom he considers to possess special qualifications for conducting such a special examination as aforesaid (in this Act referred to as a "special examination") to make the special examination.

(2) If any person who has made such a post-mortem or special examination as aforesaid is summoned by the coroner as a witness, he may be asked to give evidence as to his opinion upon any matter arising out of the examination, and as to how in his opinion the deceased came by his death.

[(3).]

115

(4) Where a person states upon oath before the coroner that in his belief the death of the deceased was caused partly or entirely by the improper or negligent treatment of a medical practitioner or other person, that medical practitioner or other person shall not be allowed to perform or assist at any post-mortem or special examination made for the purposes of the inquest on the deceased, but such medical practitoner or other person shall have the right, if he so desires, to be represented at any such post-mortem examination.

COMMENTARY ON SECTION 22

Amendments

Subsection (3) was repealed by the Coroners Act 1954, s.1 and Schedule.

SECTION 23 [Repealed]

[23.]

Notes. Section 23 was repealed by the Coroners Act 1954, s.1(2), (3) and Schedule.

SECTION 24

Power of removal of body for post-mortem examination

24.—(1) Where by the direction or at the request of a coroner a post-mortem examination of a body is to be made, the coroner may, subject as hereinafter provided, order the removal of the body to any place which may be provided for the purpose either within his jurisdiction or within any adjoining area in which another coroner has jurisdiction:

Provided that the coroner shall not under this section order the removal of the body to any place other than a place within his jurisdiction provided by a sanitary authority or nuisance authority except with the consent of the person or authority by whom the place is provided.

(2) Where a coroner orders under this section the removal of a body to any place outside his jurisdiction, he may authorize the burial of the body after examination, notwithstanding that it is outside his jurisdiction, and if he does not do so he shall order the removal of the body after examination to a place within his jurisdiction.

(3) The removal of a body in pursuance of an order made by a coroner under this section to any place outside his jurisidiction shall not affect his powers and duties in relation to the body or the inquest [touching the death of the person whose body it is], nor shall it confer or impose any rights, powers or duties upon any other coroner.

(4) The expenses of any removal ordered by a coroner under this section shall be defrayed as part of the expenses incurred by him in the course of his duties.

COMMENTARY ON SECTION 24

Amendments

In subsection (3) the words in square brackets was substituted by the Coroners Act 1980, s.1 and Schedule 1, para. 6.

SECTION 25 [Repealed]

[25.]

Note. Section 25 was repealed by The Criminal Law Act 1977, s.65 and Schedule 13.

MISCELLANEOUS AND GENERAL

SECTION 26

Power to make rules

26.—(1) The Lord Chancellor may, with the concurrence of the Secretary of State, make rules for regulating the practice and procedure at or in connection with inquests and post-mortem examinations and, in particular (without prejudice to the generality of the foregoing provision), such rules may provide—

(*a*) as to the procedure at inquests held without a jury; and

(*b*) as to the issue by coroners of orders authorizing burials; and

(*c*) for empowering a coroner or his deputy or assistant deputy to alter the date fixed for the holding of any adjourned inquest within the jurisdiction of the coroner; and

(*d*) as to the procedure to be followed where a coroner decides not to resume an adjourned inquest; and

(*e*) as to the notices to be given and as to the variation or discharge of any recognizances entered into by jurymen or witnesses where the date fixed for an adjourned inquest is altered or where a coroner decides not to resume an adjourned inquest.

[(2) Without prejudice to the generality of the preceding provisions of this section, rules under this section may make provision for persons to be excused service as jurors at inquests in such circumstances as the rules may specify.]

COMMENTARY ON SECTION 26

Amendments

Subsection (2) was added by The Coroners' Juries Act 1983, s.2.

General Note

For the rules providing for excusal from jury service see S.I. 1984 No. 552, Rules 49, 51 and 53, *ante,* at pages 57–59.

SECTION 27

Prescription of forms

27. The power of the Lord Chancellor under this Act to make rules with respect to any matter shall include power to prescribe by such rules the forms to be used in connection with that matter and to revoke or amend any forms which are directed or authorized by or under any statute to be used in connection with that matter and to substitute new forms of any of such forms.

SECTION 28

Coroners' returns

28.—(1) Section twenty-eight of the Coroners Act, 1887, under which borough coroners are required to furnish yearly returns to the Secretary of State shall apply to all other coroners in like manner as it applies to borough coroners.

(2) In addition to the yearly returns to be furnished under the said section, every coroner shall, as and when required by the Secretary of State, furnish to the Secretary of State returns in relation to inquests held and deaths inquired into by him in such form and containing such particulars as the Secretary of State may direct.

SECTION 29

Amendments as to payments to or by coroners

29.—(1) The power of a local authority under section twenty-five of the Coroners Act, 1887, to make a schedule of fees, allowances and disbursements which may lawfully be paid and made by a coroner on the holding of an inquest, shall be extended so as to permit any schedule so made to include any fees, allowances and disbursements which may lawfully be paid and made by a coroner in the course of his duties.

(2) The Secretary of State may make rules prescribing—

> (*a*) the fees payable to coroners or other persons for furnishing copies of inquisitions, depositions or other documents in their custody relating to an inquest, whether furnished under subsection (5) of section eighteen of the Coroners Act 1887, or otherwise;

(*b*) the fees, allowances and disbursements which may lawfully be paid or made by a coroner [...] where in the opinion of the Secretary of State adequate provision is not made therefor by a schedule of fees under section twenty-five of the said Act.

Amendments

In subsection (2)(*b*) the words omitted were repealed by the Coroners Act 1954, s.1(2) and Schedule.

SECTION 30

Consequential and minor amendments of the Coroners Act 1887

30. The amendments in the second column of the Second Schedule to this Act (which relate to consequential matters and to matters of minor detail) shall be made in the provisions of the Coroners Act, 1887, specified in the first column of that schedule.

SECTION 31

Repeals

31. Subject as hereinafter provided the enactments mentioned in the Third Schedule to this Act are hereby repealed to the extent specified in the third column of that schedule:

Provided that any Order in Council made under section four of the Coroners Act, 1844, shall continue in force and shall have effect as if it were an order providing for the division of a county into coroners' districts or for the alteration of an existing division of a county into coroners' districts, as the case may be, made by the Secretary of State under this Act.

SECTION 32 [Repealed]

[32.]

SECTION 33 [Repealed]

[33.]

Note. Sections 32 and 33 were repealed by The Local Government Act 1972, s.272(1) and Schedule 30.

SECTION 34

Short title, citation, construction, extent and commencement

34.—(1) This Act may be cited as the Coroners (Amendment) Act, 1926, and this Act and the Coroners Acts, 1887 and 1892, may be cited together as the Coroners Acts, 1887 to 1926.

(2) Except where the context otherwise requires, references in this Act to the Coroners Act, 1887, and to the Coroners Act, 1892, shall be construed as references to those Acts as amended by this Act and this Act shall be construed as one with those Acts.

(3) This Act shall not extend to Scotland or to Northern Ireland.

[(4).]

COMMENTARY ON SECTION 34

Amendments

Subsection (4) was repealed by the Statute Law Revision Act 1950.

FIRST SCHEDULE

Scale of Pensions. (Section 6)

1. An annual pension not exceeding ten-sixtieths of the last annual salary may be granted after the completion of a period of service of five years.

2. Where the period of service completed exceeds five years, there may be granted an annual pension not exceeding ten-sixtieths of the last annual salary, with the addition of an amount not exceeding one-fortieth of the last annual salary for each completed year's service after five years, so, however, that no such annual pension shall be of an amount exceeding two-thirds of the last annual salary.

3. For the purposes of this schedule the last annual salary of a coroner shall be taken to be the salary paid to him in respect of his last completed year of service as coroner, after deducting so much if any of that salary as was paid to the coroner with a view to his providing at his own expense for any necessary expenditure in connection with his duties as coroner, and if any dispute arises as to the amount to be deducted under this paragraph in computing the salary of a coroner the dispute shall be referred to the Secretary of State whose decision thereon shall be final and conclusive.

Note. See S.I. 1978 No. 374.

THE CORONERS ACT 1954

(2 & 3 Eliz. 2, c. 31)

An Act to amend the law as to the fees and allowances payable by coroners to witnesses, to persons summoned to attend as witnesses and to medical practitioners making post mortem examinations by the coroner's direction or at the coroner's request.

[June 4, 1954]

SECTION 1

Fees and expenses of witnesses and doctors to be regulated by rules of Secretary of State

1. (1) The fees and allowances which may be lawfully paid by coroners—

    (*a*) to witnesses and persons summoned to attend as witnesses; and

    (*b*) to medical practitioners making post mortem examinations by the coroner's direction or at the coroner's request,

shall, instead of being such as are or may be prescribed by or under section twenty-five of the Coroners Act, 1887, or section twenty-three or paragraph (*b*) of subsection (2) of section twenty-nine of the Coroners (Amendment) Act, 1926, be such as may be prescribed by rules to be made under this subsection (by statutory instrument) by the Secretary of State:

Provided that the preceding provisions of this subsection shall not affect the fees payable in respect of any such special examination of parts or contents of the body or other substances or things as is mentioned in paragraph (*b*) of subsection (1) of section twenty-two of the Coroners (Amendment) Act, 1926, and accordingly the fees in respect of any such special examination made at the request of the coroner under that section shall be such as may be prescribed by the Schedule made by the local authority under the said section twenty-five or by the rules, if any, made by the Secretary of State under paragraph (*b*) of subsection (2) of the said section twenty-nine.

(2) The enactments mentioned in the Schedule to this Act are hereby repealed to the extent specified in the third column of that Schedule.

(3) This Act shall come into force on such day as the Secretary of State may by order (which shall be a statutory instrument) appoint and nothing in this Act shall affect any fees or allowances paid before that day.

(4) Any increase attributable to the passing of this Act in the sums which under Part I of the Local Government Act, 1948, or under the Local Government (Financial Provisions) (Scotland) Act, 1954, are payable out of moneys provided by Parliament shall be defrayed out of moneys so provided.

COMMENTARY ON SECTION 1

General Note

The Administration of Justice Act 1977 made fees and expenses of witnesses and doctors determinable administratively by the Secretary of State with the consent of the minister for the Civil Service, instead of being prescribed by Rules.

The provisions governing allowances payable to jurors are set out in the 1926 Act, s.25A.

THE CORONERS ACT 1980

(c. 38)

An Act to abolish the obligation of coroners under the law of England and Wales to view the bodies on which they hold inquests; to make fresh provision for inquests to be held in districts other than that in which the body lies; to confer new powers for the exhumation of bodies; and for connected purposes.

[July 17, 1980]

SECTION 1

Abolition of requirement for a coroner holding an inquest to view the body

1. It shall not be obligatory for a coroner holding an inquest on a body to view the body and—

- (*a*) the validity of an inquest shall not be questioned in any court on the ground that the coroner did not view the body;
- (*b*) the enactments specified in Schedule 1 and Schedule 2 to this Act (which relate to the view of the body by the coroner and jury) are amended or repealed as provided in those Schedules; and
- (*c*) no body shall be ordered by a coroner to be exhumed except under section 4 of this Act.

SECTION 2

Power to hold inquests in areas other than that in which the body lies

2.—(1) If it appears to a coroner that an inquest ought to be held on a body lying within his area but it is expedient that the inquest should be held by some other coroner he may request that coroner to assume jurisdiction to hold the inquest and if that coroner agrees he, and not the coroner within whose area the body is lying, shall have jurisdiction to hold the inquest.

(2) If the coroner who has been requested to assume jurisdiction declines to assume it the coroner who has made the request may apply to the Secretary of State for a direction designating the coroner who is to hold the inquest.

(3) On the making of an application under subsection (2) above the Secretary of State shall determine by which coroner (whether one of the two mentioned in that subsection or another) the inquest should in all the circumstances be held and shall direct him to assume jurisdiction or, as the case may be, to exercise his jurisdiction to hold the inquest; and where a

direction is given under this subsection directing a coroner to assume jurisdiction he, and not the coroner within whose area the body is lying, shall have jurisdiction to hold the inquest and shall hold it accordingly.

(4) Where jurisdiction to hold an inquest is assumed under this section it shall not be necessary to remove the body into the area of the coroner who is to hold the inquest.

(5) Any request made or agreement given, any application for a direction and any direction under any of the preceding provisions of this section shall be made or given in writing.

(6) Notice of the making of an application by one coroner under subsection (2) above shall be given to the other coroner and notice of the direction given pursuant to it shall be given, in a case where the direction is given to the coroner who has made or the coroner who had notice of the application, to the other coroner and, in a case where the direction is given to some other coroner, to the coroner who made and the coroner who had notice of the application.

SECTION 3

Provisions supplementary to s.2

3.—(1) On the assumption by a coroner of jurisdiction to hold an inquest under section 2 above that coroner shall also assume, in relation to the body and the inquest, all the powers and duties which would belong to him if the body were lying within his area (including the power to order its exhumation under section 4 below) and may exercise those powers notwithstanding that the body remains outside his area or, having been removed into it, is removed out of it by virtue of any order of his for its examination or burial.

(2) On the assumption of the powers and duties referred to in subsection (1) above by the coroner who assumes jurisdiction to hold the inquest the coroner within whose area the body is lying shall cease to have any powers or duties in relation to the body or the inquest notwithstanding that the body remains within his area or comes to be buried there.

(3) It shall be for the coroner who assumes, and not for the coroner who ceases to have, jurisdiction to hold an inquest under section 2 above to pay any fees or other expenses incurred in the course of his duties by the latter coroner before he ceased to have jurisdiction and such fees and expenses shall be accounted for and repaid accordingly.

(4) At the beginning of section 7(1) of the Coroners Act 1887 (jurisdiction of a coroner dependent on the presence of the body in his area) there shall be inserted the words "Unless he has assumed jurisdiction under section 2 of the Coroners Act 1980."

(5) Sections 16 and 17 of the Coroners (Amendment) Act 1926 (which are superseded by section 2 above and this section) are hereby repealed.

123

SECTION 4

Power of coroner to order exhumation of bodies

4.—(1) A coroner may order the exhumation of the body of a person buried within the area within which he has jurisdiction where it appears to him that it is necessary for the body to be examined—

> (*a*) for the purpose of his holding an inquest touching that person's death or discharging any other function of his in relation to the body or the death; or
>
> (*b*) for the purposes of any criminal proceedings which have been instituted or are contemplated in respect of the death of that person or of some other person who came by his death in circumstances connected with the death of the person whose body is needed for examination.

(2) The power of a coroner under this section shall be exercisable by warrant under his hand.

SECTION 5

Citation, construction and extent

5.—(1) This Act may be cited as the Coroners Act 1980 and shall be construed as one with the Coroners Acts 1887 to 1954 and those Acts and this Act may be cited together as the Coroners Acts 1887 to 1980.

(2) This Act extends to England and Wales only except that the repeal in section 30(2)(*a*) of the Merchant Shipping Act 1979 extends also to Northern Ireland.

SCHEDULE 1

CONSEQUENTIAL AMENDMENTS

The Coroners Act 1887

1. In section 3(2) of the Coroners Act 1887, for the words "on the body", there shall be substituted the words "touching the death".

2. In section 29(4) of the said Act of 1887, for the word "body" in the second place where it occurs, there shall be substituted the word "person".

The Coroners (Amendment) Act 1926

3. In section 13(1) of the Coroners (Amendment) Act 1926, for the words "on the body", there shall be substituted the words "into the death of that person".

4. In section 18 of the said Act of 1926, for the words from "held otherwise" to "lying", there shall be substituted the words "one into the death of a person whose body does not lie".

5. In section 20(8) of the said Act of 1926, for the words "upon the body", there shall be substituted the words "touching the death".

6. In section 21(1) of the said Act of 1926, for the words "upon the body", there shall be substituted the words "touching the death".

7. In section 24(3) of the said Act of 1926, for the word "thereon", there shall be substituted the words "touching the death of the person whose body it is".

INDEX

127